WHAT PEOPLE

CRYSTAL PI

This book is a thoughtful exploration of the chakra system for those who wish to support their spiritual development with the practical use of crystals. It is heartening to see many minor chakras included, as folks tend to forget that there are hundreds of chakras, not just the well-known six or seven! Included, too, is some well-researched guidance on kundalini, a topic that can appear glamorous and appealing to some, and a reality of dissonance and discomfort to those in whom it activates without appropriate support. Full of good advice giving a balanced overview of a complex and fascinating subject. Judy emphasises a grounded and practical approach tailored to individual need, useful for both beginners and the more experienced.

Simon and Sue Lilly, authors of *Crystal Healing* (Watkins•
Books) and *The Illustrated Elements of Crystal Healing*

This is one of those books that you will always keep and dip back into. I recommend this for any therapist or person who wishes to explore the deeper intuitive side of the chakra system and the kundalini energy. The understanding of emotional anatomy in connection to our energy centres and fields give a deeper result to healing. Learning how to embrace and understand the power of the kundalini energy which quite frankly is wasted by 90% of us, will elevate you to a higher level of consciousness. You won't want to put this mine of information down.

Sarah Lownds, Founder of Sarpenela Natural Therapies Centre. www.sarpenela.co.uk

Judy Hall is truly a master of her subject; she brings us a vast wealth of knowledge and research combined with her accessible and engaging delivery. In these times of shifting consciousness, Judy's timely book guides us in how to assimilate the higher dimensional frequencies that have opened and bring them into our everyday life, supported by the appropriate tried and tested crystals.

Gill Matini, Principal, College of Psychic Studies

CRYSTAL
PRESCRIPTIONS

Volume 4

The A-Z guide to
chakra balancing crystals and
kundalini activation stones

Volumes in this series

Crystal Prescriptions volume 1: The A-Z guide to over 1,200 symptoms and their healing crystals

Crystal Prescriptions volume 2: The A-Z guide to over 1,250 conditions and their new generation healing crystals

Crystal Prescriptions volume 3: Crystal solutions to electro-magnetic pollution and geopathic stress. An A-Z guide.

Crystal Prescriptions volume 4: The A-Z guide to chakra balancing crystals and kundalini activation stones

Crystal Prescriptions volume 5: Space clearing, Feng Shui and Psychic Protection. An A-Z guide.

Crystal Prescriptions volume 6: Crystals for ancestral clearing, soul retrieval, spirit release and karmic healing. An A-Z guide.

Crystal Prescriptions volume 7: The A-Z Guide to Creating Crystal Essences for Abundant Well-Being, Environmental Healing and Astral-Magic

CRYSTAL
PRESCRIPTIONS

Volume 4

The A-Z guide to
chakra balancing crystals and
kundalini activation stones

Judy Hall

Author of the best-selling

The Crystal Bible series

BOOKS

Winchester, UK
Washington, USA

JOHN HUNT PUBLISHING

First published by O-Books, 2015
O-Books is an imprint of John Hunt Publishing Ltd., 3 East St., Alresford,
Hampshire SO24 9EE, UK
office@jhpbooks.com
www.johnhuntpublishing.com
www.o-books.com

For distributor details and how to order please visit the 'Ordering' section on our
website.

ISBN: 978 1 78535 053 5
978 1 78535 054 2 (ebook)

A CIP catalogue record for this book is available from the British Library.

Design: Stuart Davies

UK: Printed and bound by CPI Group (UK) Ltd, Croydon, CR0 4YY
Printed in North America by CPI GPS partners

We operate a distinctive and ethical publishing philosophy
in all areas of our business, from our global network of
authors to production and worldwide distribution.

CONTENTS

Disclaimer

The information given in this directory is in no way intended to be a substitute for treatment by a medical practitioner. Further assistance can also be sought from a suitably qualified crystal healing or kundalini yoga practitioner. Healing can be defined as bringing the body, emotions, mind and spirit back into balance. It does not imply a cure.

Acknowledgements

My deepest thanks to *shaman extraordinaire* Sarah Lownds of Sarpenela Natural Therapies (www.sarpenela .co.uk) for joining up the dots that led to kundalini flow. Thanks are due also to all the workshop participants and clients who taught me so much about the chakras, expanded consciousness, and kundalini awakening – and its side effects. Their willingness to follow where I led into uncharted territory to explore new crystals and chakras, and the higher dimensions, made this book possible.

And I must add my grateful thanks to Terrie Birch, astrologer and wise woman, for giving up her lunch break to take the cover photograph. Many blessings to you.

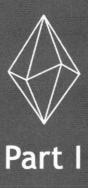

Part I

Introduction

The Dance of Shakti and Shiva

Kundalini is the mass explosion of dark, raw, sexual, moist, sticky, juicy power. It is distinctly the wild feminine which can't be controlled. It is primitive, messy and overpowering, like birth and can be as frightening as death.
– Dr Glenn Morris
(www.kundaliniawakeningprocess.com)

Have you experienced a firestorm rushing up your spine? Electric shocks or tingles coursing through your body? Waves of energy flowing through you like ripples on the sea? Or icy chills? An instantaneous cosmic orgasm? A 'scintillation of the senses'? Ultimate bliss? Momentary enlightenment? Being bathed in liquid light? Or been blasted out of your body? If so, you've had a kundalini event.

If not, if you've picked up this book you might well be seeking such an experience. Or soliciting ascension. Kundalini goes by many names. But, you may be afraid of what you'll encounter when you do. There are many warnings out there about this mysterious, overwhelming force that can rush up your spine and fountain out of your head. Authentic empowerment is on offer. But not without its Pooh-traps and peccadilloes, as we'll see. I particularly like the quote above as for me it encapsulates the core experience of fiery kundalini awakening. The wildness of the Shakti force – primordial cosmic energy – moving through you to meld with the pure primal consciousness of Shiva and give birth to expanded awareness.

This book approaches kundalini and the chakras through a Western energetic-healing frame of reference. I don't claim to be an expert in kundalini but I have encountered it many times in various guises over the last 45 years. I've worked with crystals to cleanse and activate the traditional and 'newer' chakras, and facilitate the smooth rising of power throughout the physical and subtle energy bodies. I've used crystals to ameliorate adverse side effects of kundalini, without necessarily attributing them to kundalini activation. But which, with the benefit of hindsight, I have come to recognize as exactly that. I have also learned a great deal about the high vibrational chakras, their blockages and place in expanded awareness and spiritual evolution during that time. I'd like to share the fruits of my experience with you.

Where crystals really come into their own is in bringing about a vibrational shift of consciousness, literally taking us into a new dimension – or rather opening all possible dimensions. There are many crystals available now whose aim is to usher in awareness and integrate the perception of being both human and divine at the same time. Historically, this has been described as the Dance of Shakti (power) and Shiva (unadulterated consciousness). Raising awareness and linking with the divine has always been the aim of kundalini activation. But the crystals point out that we cannot achieve this unity until we have completed our personal healing and growth work – and prepared our chakras to mediate the energetic flow. Kundalini rising can stimulate a cleansing catharsis as the energies shift. This shift can be assisted by preliminary chakra work, including opening the higher chakras, and raising the kundalini in gentle, purifying stages. So, in this book you'll find all the preparatory information you need on the chakras, old and new, what blocks and clears them and the physio-logical, psychological and spiritual effect they can have.

Then we move on to kundalini. No longer a secret teaching shared only with initiates, considerable attention is now being given to raising the kundalini force, and scientists are becoming interested in researching the effects. This subtle but extremely dynamic psycho-spiritual energy can irradiate the cells of our physical and etheric bodies with a new resonance. One that literally en-light-ens us. That is, it awakens our lightbody and our ability to assimilate higher dimen-sional frequencies. But unless this is done with due care the rise may be uncontrolled with unexpected consequences including immense discomfort. The best way to ensure that the rise is under your control is to have all your chakras open and functioning at optimum, the subtle energy bodies in harmony, *and to use crystals to mediate the flow.*

Preparation for raising kundalini includes activating some of the lesser known and the higher vibration chakras such as the causal vortex, which give access to expanded awareness of the multidimensional reality all around us. Higher consciousness and multidimensional realities cannot be explored unless you are well grounded through the earth star and Gaia gateway, however. Whilst much attention has been paid to the major, conventional seven chakras, the lesser known chakras are vital to kundalini assimilation and fully utilising your healing and intuitive abilities. Energy work or Reiki, for instance, is greatly enhanced by opening the palm chakras. Research conducted in Japan, for example, demonstrated that practitioners of healing and martial arts techniques were capable of emanating extraordinarily large and strong pulsating magnetic fields from the palms of their hands many times stronger than normal human biomagnetic fields.[1]

Similarly, you can only be power-full if you have activated and filled your dantien. Opening the earth star beneath your feet and the knee chakras help you to anchor the energy into everyday reality. Opening the Gaia gateway links you into higher dimension and divine connections and then grounds them. Until all the chakras have been activated, kundalini cannot be fully assimilated and will simply shoot out from the top of the head, or, worse, leak from your base chakra downwards. According to where its passage has been blocked, it can also spread out sideways to affect your physiology, psychology and psyche.

Throughout this book we will be using tried and tested crystals to cleanse and activate essential chakra connections, to harmonize the subtle energy bodies, and to mediate higher dimensional energies to prepare the way for kundalini initiation.

What is a Chakra?

The chakras or force-centres are points of connection at which energy flows from one vehicle or body of a man to another... When quite undeveloped they appear as small circles about two inches in diameter, glowing dully... but when awakened and vivified they are seen as blazing, coruscating whirlpools, much increased in size, and resembling miniature suns.
– CW Leadbeater

The chakras are multilayered, multidimensional vortexes of subtle energy that radiate several feet out from your physical body. Linkage points between the physical and subtle energy bodies, they are metaphysical rather than physical but they are essential to our efficient functioning in the world and to raising our consciousness. The Sanskrit word means 'wheel' but they act more like a vortex or valve, regulating the flow of energy through the subtle and physical bodies via the meridian, endocrine and nervous systems. They mediate how much energy and what feelings you take in from the world around you, and your response to that outer world. Loosely speaking, the chakras below the waist are primarily physical, although they can affect the endocrine glands and from that the personality. Those in the upper torso are aligned to emotional functioning that can create psychosomatic conditions, as can those in the head that function on a mental and intuitive basis but which may have physical repercussions.

The chakras are an ancient concept that appears in many philosophies. Ancient Hindu texts speak of them as do early Egyptian writings. These texts reveal a deep understanding of the effect of the chakras and subtle energy on the body-mind through the endocrine system. An understanding which modern scientists are only just catching up with in their research into the effects of melatonin, picoline, serotonin and DMT. The secretions of the brain that govern metaphysical as well as physical functioning. As Serena Roney-Dougal, who has been researching such connections for many years, puts it:

> Our knowledge of the endocrine system, the chemistry of our body-mind and emotional system, is still meagre... However, partial as our knowledge may be, it does fit together with what the yogis, 'scientists of the subtle mind', tell us about the yogic chakra system. Our disciplines, apparently so different in language and method, appear to corroborate each other.
> – Serena Roney-Dougal

How active your chakras are and whether they are stressed or functioning at optimum powerfully affects your perceptions and your emotions, and how you express your inner world. If they are 'bunged up', they allow subconscious fears and feelings to rule unchallenged. If they are operating well, they test and challenge perceptions and experiences rather than blindly

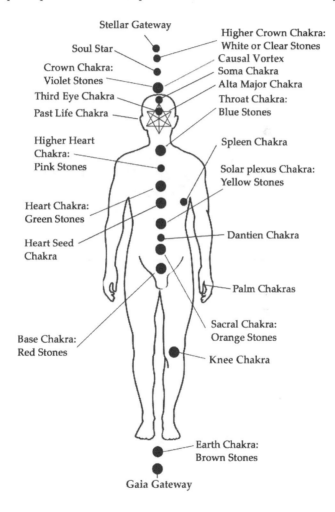

Stellar Gateway

Soul Star

Crown Chakra:
Violet Stones

Third Eye Chakra

Past Life Chakra

Higher Heart
Chakra:
Pink Stones

Heart Chakra:
Green Stones

Heart Seed
Chakra

Base Chakra:
Red Stones

Higher Crown Chakra:
White or Clear Stones
Causal Vortex
Soma Chakra
Alta Major Chakra
Throat Chakra:
Blue Stones

Spleen Chakra

Solar plexus Chakra:
Yellow Stones

Dantien Chakra

Palm Chakras

Sacral Chakra:
Orange Stones

Knee Chakra

Earth Chakra:
Brown Stones

Gaia Gateway

following the same old pathway. This is why the chakras are so important in human and soul evolution. They assist in assimilating downloads of higher vibrational energy that lift the soul beyond what has been known before.

The chakras have an essential part to play in well-being at every level. Each chakra 'governs' an area of life and an organ or part of the body, and has to do with specific thoughts and emotions. Stress, tension,

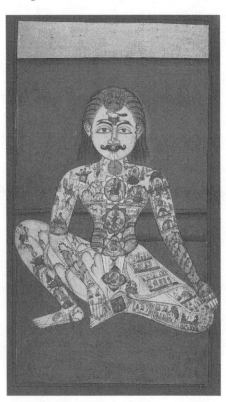

distortion or sluggishness in a chakra will ultimately manifest as dis-ease within the physical body, or be reflected in psychosomatic or psychological distress. Restore the equilibrium and rebalance the chakra, and the dis-ease or distress disappears.

Chakra healing

Traditionally, each chakra is linked to specific organs and has its own colour, although, as we will see, there are also other differently coloured crystals that relate to the chakras. It is a question of resonance and harmony rather than simply colour. Certain crystals will stimulate a sluggish chakra, others will slow down an overactive one – the directory has a comprehensive list. If a chakra is spinning too rapidly or is stuck open, using a complementary coloured crystal from the colour wheel (see page 29) can bring it back to equilibrium. Simply select a crystal of a colour from the opposite side of the wheel to the traditional chakra colour. Then dowse to check that it will work for you. A crystal of the same traditional colour as the chakra will stimulate a sluggish or blocked spin. By placing crystals of the *appropriate* colour and vibration on the chakras, chakra imbalances are quickly eliminated and the chakras harmonized to work together, leading to better health and a sense of well-being.

Chakra spin

The chakras whirl and it is not so much the direction of

spin that matters but rather the speed *and whether it is an appropriate direction for the individual.* Each person has a direction of spin that is right for them, which can be checked by dowsing. Occasionally the direction of spin needs to be reversed but more often it is the rate that needs adjusting. Whether a chakra is open or closed affects how energy flows through it, but so too does the speed of rotation. If a chakra is spinning slowly it will be sluggish and blocked, deficient in energy, so that it cannot mediate flow or receive fresh input. If it is spinning too rapidly then it is stuck open and energy will be whirling in and out without restraint. Crystals adjust the rate – and direction – of spin to optimum, and assist with opening and closing the chakras as appropriate.

If a chakra is stuck open and spinning too fast, this may be because the chakras above and/or below it have blockages and are stagnant and toxic so that energy cannot circulate freely along the spine and through the subtle bodies. So those chakras would also need treating. The aim is to have all the chakras balanced and functioning at optimum.

Blown or blocked chakra

If a chakra is stuck open and spinning too fast, it is known as a blown chakra. A blown chakra is particularly vulnerable to outside influence as there is no protection or mediation of the energy flow. A blown chakra may be quite literally 'blown away', that is, out of line with the other chakras. If when dowsing or checking how chakra energy is flowing it veers off towards one or other sides of the body, then the chakra will need bringing back into line. That is, it needs to be aligned not only in spin and energetic frequency with the other chakras but also moved back into vertical alignment.

Similarly, a chakra can be stuck in the closed position – and energy may divert around it. Deficient in energy, a blocked chakra leads to blockages and negative qualities manifesting. A chakra may be blocked because of your own past input, conscious or otherwise, or because other people 'put a block' on it – that is they seek to control you, don't want you to see something, and so on. Chakra blockages have many issues and it pays to search for the deeper cause.

What blocks a chakra?

There are many reasons why a chakra may become blocked or blown, and to some extent this depends on where the chakra is situated along the line. Geopathic stress, electromagnetic pollution and too long spent under artificial rather than natural light has a profound effect on the physical body and its associated chakras. But old traumas, toxicity, close-mindedness and fixed beliefs, emotional pain and physical injuries can all contribute. They become an energetic pattern or engram that is imprinted into the appropriate chakra or subtle energy body at a very deep level. However, one of the major causes of blocked or blown chakras is past life issues that have been carried over into the present life.

The directory covers crystals to remedy a wide range of these past life causes (see page 301). These issues are imprinted in the karmic subtle energy body and the past life and causal vortex chakras. The layers may need to be peeled back gently over a period of time until the core issue is reached. It can then be released and the energy transmuted.

Chakra Colours

What we perceive as colour is simply the brain's way of recognizing the many different energy qualities of light. Every frequency of visible light, each colour, creates change in us at many different levels: physically, emotionally and mentally.
– Sue and Simon Lilly, *Healing with Crystals and Chakra Energies*

Colour arises from the splitting of light. It is an energetic vibration and is perceived by receptors in the brain, or with a psychic eye. Each colour ray has a subtle effect physiologically, psychologically and spiritually. While colour seems to have long been associated with the chakras, both historically and in the modern day there is little consensus on the actual chakra colours. The 'traditional' colours are comparatively modern attributions and many older chakra drawings show a completely different range of colours. This lack of consensus is particularly striking with regard to the 'newer', higher dimension chakras, many of which are also shown on older chakra illustrations. This is because each body has a slight variation in frequency and so the resonance of the colour – and the crystals attributed to a chakra – will affect each person in a subtly dissimilar way. You may perceive a somewhat altered colour spectrum as your higher faculties open. Many people report that colours become more luminous, pulsating, almost incandescent, and may be beyond the familiar spectrum so that description is difficult.

Chakra	Colour
Earth Star	brown, dark grey, maroon
Knee	multicoloured, tan
Base	red
Sacral	orange
Dantien	reddish-orange, amber
Solar Plexus	yellow, light greenish yellow
Spleen	green
Heart Seed	pale pearlescent blue, pink, white
Heart	green/pink
Higher Heart	pink, gold, purple, blue
Palm	silver-white, golden-white, red, blue
Throat	blue, turquoise
Third Eye	indigo
Soma	blue, lavender, white, ultra-violet
Crown	white, purple, lavender
Stellar Gateway	deep violet, white, gold, silver or clear

Soul Star	magenta, white, black
Alta Major	magenta, green
Causal Vortex	white, gold
Gaia Gateway	black, brown, silver, gold

The Colour Wheel

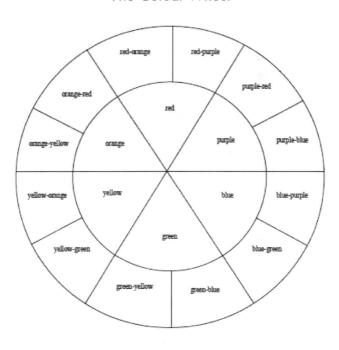

Created for Modern Handmade Child by Hi Mamma

The Personal Chakras

Every thought and experience you've ever had in your life gets filtered through these chakra databases. Each event is recorded into your cells.
– Caroline Myss

The personal chakras govern the sphere of everyday reality and how you react or respond to the world around you – although they may be a knee-jerk reaction to inner states of being such as emotions or habits. Mediating between the inner and outer worlds, and your physical body and the energies of Earth, they assist in assimilating energies and frequencies at the lower level of the scale. They also affect how well or otherwise your body, emotions and mind function. Roughly speaking, the chakras in the belly correspond to the physical level of being, those in the upper torso to the emotional and from the throat upwards into the skull the mental level. Chakras above the head work mainly at the spiritual level. They work in conjunction with the subtle auric bodies that are closest in frequency to those levels of being. Although there are many chakras, including the lesser known (pages 56–74), seven major personal chakras are traditionally utilised. But, to this must be added an eighth, the earth star which is essential for keeping you grounded and in touch with the Earth whilst in incarnation.

Traditionally the organs, systems and endocrinology of the physical body have been linked with specific chakras, all of which you will find under the individual chakra entries in the first half of this book. Each chakra is also connected to a sense. The senses range from those of touch, sight and so on, through more subtle senses such as safety and security, to the metaphysics of inner sight and spiritual connection. Imbalances or blockages, rapid or sluggish spin cycles in a chakra relating to an organ, gland or sense will, ultimately, have a physical effect. Crystal healing is based on the premise that placing an appropriate stone on the chakra restores it to balance and the problem then stabilizes itself.

The chakras are not static. Like the whole human organism, they have the capacity to evolve. Crystals assist in opening higher, finer and more subtle layers and levels of the personal chakras as well as the subtle energy bodies, and reactivating dormant higher chakras. They then integrate and ground the interconnected system to bring higher dimensional energies into everyday reality. You become an expression of those expanded vibrations. To facilitate this, there are energetic connective correspondences between the personal and the higher chakras. These are listed under relevant chakras.

The Earth Star Chakra

The sphere of everyday reality and groundedness

Location: About a foot beneath the feet.

The earth star chakra connects you to the Earth's core as well as its electromagnetic fields and energy meridians. This chakra helps you to bring things into concrete form, grounding and anchoring new frequencies and actualising your plans and dreams. It is a place of safety and regeneration. Without it, you will have only a toehold in incarnation and be physically and psychologically ungrounded. With it, you have a stable, calm and strong centre from which to handle the vicissitudes of life and its pleasures with equal composure. If your earth star is not functioning well you will be unable to assimilate and ground kundalini energy when it is awakened. When the chakra is functioning at optimum you have a natural electrical circuit providing a physical and spiritual energy boost. The sciatic nerve, the longest nerve in the body, runs from the heel of the foot up the legs to the hips and then across and into the spine. Passing up the spine it connects your brain to the vibrations of the Earth. It also connects your earth star chakra with the knee chakras and those chakras to the base so that you are fully grounded and connected to the physical dimension of being.

Physiology: The physical body, electrical and meridian systems of the body, sciatic nerve and the sensory organs.

Sense: Security and survival.

Positive quality: Empowerment. When this chakra is functioning well you are grounded and comfortable in incarnation with a well-functioning immune system and the ability to anchor higher dimensional energies into the earth plane. You will be practical and operate well in everyday reality but will be open to assimilating higher dimensional energies.

Negative quality: Powerlessness and ungroundedness.

Higher chakra correspondence: The soul star chakra.

Overactive/blown/spin too fast: If your earth star is blown you will lack grounding and have no connection to the planet or awareness of being part of a greater overall system. Or, paradoxically, you may be overly concerned for the planet and not give enough attention to your own body. An out of balance earth star easily picks up adverse environmental factors such as geopathic stress and toxic pollutants. It is highly sensitive to electromagnetic energy as it governs the electrical systems of the body and is your connection to the planet through the soles of your feet with their many nerve endings and minor chakras.

Underactive/blocked/spin too slow: Earth star blockages or disruptions lead to discomfort in your physical body, a sense of not belonging on the planet. With little body awareness, there are feelings of helplessness and ungroundedness accompanied by an inability to function practically in the world. You will be unable to assimilate higher dimensional energies.

Typical dis-eases are lethargic: ME, arthritis, cancer, muscular disorders, depression, psychiatric disturbances, autoimmune diseases, persistent tiredness.

Attachments: Spirits of place, stuck spirits. If this chakra is permanently open, you can easily pick up negative energies from the ground or 'spirits of place', either as attachments or as a communication of events that have taken place.

Opening the earth star and the grounding root

Keeping your earth star chakra open and grounded into the centre of the planet helps you to be comfortable in incarnation and facilitates assimilation of higher dimensional and kundalini energies. As this chakra is so important, we're going to break off here to open it. The simplest way to do this is with a visualization assisted by a crystal:

- Stand with your feet slightly apart, well balanced on your knees and hips. Feet flat on the floor. Place a Flint, Eye of the Storm (Judy's Jasper), Graphic Smoky Quartz, Hematite, Smoky Quartz, Smoky Elestial Quartz or other grounding stone at your feet.
- Picture the earth star chakra about a foot beneath your feet opening like the petals of a water lily.
- Feel two roots growing from the soles of your feet down to meet at the earth star.
- The two roots twine together and pass down

through the earth star going deep into the Earth. They pass through the outer mantle, down past the solid crust and deep into the molten magma.

- When the entwined roots have passed through the magma, they reach the big iron crystal ball at the centre of the planet.
- The roots hook themselves around this ball, holding you firmly in incarnation and helping you to be grounded in incarnation.
- Energy and protection can flow up this root to keep you energized and safe.
- Allow the roots to pass up from the earth star through your feet, up your legs and the knee chakras and into your hips. At your hips the roots move across to meet in the base chakra and from there to the sacral and the dantien. The energy that flows up from the centre of the Earth can be stored in the dantien (see page 64).

Note: Whenever you are in an area of seriously disturbed Earth energy, protect your earth star chakra by visualizing a large protective crystal all around it. The root will still be able to pass down to the centre of the Earth to bring powerful energy to support you, and the crystal will help to transmute and stabilize the negative energy. A virtual crystal can work when visualized with intent, but placing an actual crystal here intensifies the effect. *See also the shamanic and cosmic anchor exercise on page 115.*

The Base/Root Chakra (Muladhara)

The sphere of basic survival instincts and security issues

Location: Base of your spine, tailbone, coccyx, perineum. The Sanskrit name for this chakra means 'root support'. Your base chakra is linked to your core energy and to your connection to Earth. It is the foundation for all the other chakras along the spine, a secure base on which they rest. It represents both your home and your career: your place in the world. When it functions well you are grounded and connected to your core. It is where the kundalini force lies curled around your tailbone before it is awakened. The base chakra is also the area of the will to survive and the ability to make things happen. This is where you discover yourself as an individual and take responsibility for yourself. It is where you recognize the tribe to which you belong and where you feel safe. When this chakra is functioning well, you trust the universe. Imbalances here lead to sexual disturbances and feelings of stuckness, anger, impotence and frustration – and the inability to let go. The fight or flight response is permanently activated with resultant dis-ease.

Physiology: The 'fight or flight' response, adrenals, bladder, elimination systems, gonads, immune system, kidneys, lower back, lower extremities, sciatic nerve, lymph system, prostate gland, rectum, skeletal system (teeth and bones), veins.

Sense: Smell, trust and survival instinct.

Positive quality: Inner security and connectedness.

When this chakra is functioning well you are confident and self-assertive, and able to deal effectively with environmental stresses.

Negative quality: Insecurity and alienation. If the base chakra is affected by geopathic stress or toxic electromagnetic fields your immune system cannot protect you. Imbalances or disruption in this chakra lead to insecurity and feelings of anger, impotence and frustration.

Higher chakra correspondence: The causal vortex.

Overactive/blown/spin too fast: When this chakra is racing flat out it is easy to become sexually obsessed, continually seeking satisfaction 'out there' rather than making an inner connection and developing personality traits that will sustain you. This can lead to alcohol, drug and other addictive or comfort-seeking behaviour. You will be floaty, ungrounded, and may experience uncontrolled out-of-body experiences, dark sexual fantasies and vivid dreams.

Underactive/blocked/spin too slow: When this chakra is blocked you will feel impotent and may become physically so. Lacking bioenergetic balance, you will be ungrounded and may be unwilling to accept your connection to the Earth, feeling uncomfortable in your physical body and seeking escape. It leads to feelings of isolation and alienation and, at the extreme, to fantasies of self-destruction.

Typical dis-eases are constant, low level or flare up suddenly and may reflect disconnection from the Earth:

Stiffness or tingling in joints, poor circulation in the lower limbs, sciatica, chronic lower back pain, renal, reproductive or rectal disorders such as fluid retention or constipation (diarrhoea if stuck open), prostate problems, haemorrhoids, varicose veins or hernias, the extremes of bipolar disorder, addictions, glandular disturbances, personality and anxiety disorders, skeletal/bone/teeth problems, autoimmune diseases. Insomnia and disturbed sleep is common, as is waking up tired and unrefreshed.

Attachments: Previous partners, your children, anyone you've ever had sex with, needy people, thought forms, parents particularly the mother, unborn children, miscarriages and stillbirths. Previous partners or significant others leave their imprint in these chakras and can continue to influence through the association.

The Sacral/Navel Chakra (Svadisthana)
The sphere of creativity, passion and fertility
Location: About a hand's breadth below your waist, just below the navel.

The Sanskrit name for this chakra means 'one's own base'. This creative chakra is an important part of your core energy system and affects your ability to bring things into manifestation. It also assists you to hold your boundaries steady. It has a great deal to do with how you handle your immediate environment and matters such as money, career and authority figures. When this chakra is working well you experience yourself as a dynamic agent of change in your life. If it is blocked you cannot experience yourself as a potent sexual being, causing feelings of impotence and powerlessness. If it is blown, you will be subjected to overwhelming sexual urges. This chakra affects how easily you express your sexuality and how you feel about relationships. It may also hold on to parenting issues and the connection to your family. Imbalances here lead to infertility and blocked creativity at all levels. The sacral chakra is where 'hooks' from other people may make themselves felt, particularly from previous sexual encounters. This is one of the 'pleasure chakras' that enlivens life by stimulating the production of endorphins and 'feel good' hormones so it has a powerful effect on how you feel from moment to moment. When this chakra is functioning well you are able to give and receive in equal measure. When it is not, you may feel shut off from nurturing and sharing, or feel jealous and possessive.

Physiology: Bladder and gallbladder, immune and elimination systems, kidneys, large and small intestine, lumbar and pelvic region, sacrum, spleen, ovaries, testes, uterus.

Sense: Taste, sensations, appetite.

Positive quality: Self-worth and confidence. When it is functioning well you are creative and enlivened.

Negative quality: Selfish with low self-esteem.

Chakra connection: Throat.

Overactive/blown/spin too fast: When this chakra is wide open you may experience urinary tract and bladder problems as the organs of elimination are constantly overstimulated. There will be no filter on sexual urges, libido will be high and out of control, but frustration may occur at all levels.

Underactive/blocked/spin too slow: When this chakra is blocked you may experience chronic lower back or sciatic pain, gynaecological problems and pelvic pain. This chakra being blocked typically leads to sexual problems in both men and women. Psychologically, you may feel that you are 'not good enough'. This may cause you to cling to what you have in an effort to gain more affection. It may also cause you to underachieve in your chosen career.

Typical dis-eases are toxic and psychosomatic: PMT and muscle cramps, sciatica, reproductive blockages or diseases, prostate problems, impotence, infertility, fibroids, endometriosis, allergies, addictions, eating disorders, diabetes, liver or intestinal dysfunction, irritable bowel syndrome, chronic back pain, urinary infections.

Attachments: Previous partners, children, anyone you've ever had sexual relations with (whether physical or in the mind), needy people, thought forms, parents particularly the mother, unborn children, miscarriages and stillbirths. Previous partners or significant others leave their imprint in this chakra and can continue to influence through the association.

The Solar Plexus Chakra (Manipura)

The sphere of emotional communication and assimilation

Location: Hand's breadth above the waist.

The Sanskrit name for this chakra means 'jewelled city'. It is where you store your emotions, and it can have a profoundly psychosomatic effect. Your feelings are reflected in your dis-eases – and your speech. 'Feeling gutted' for example feels as though there is a hollowness in this chakra, and gut problems as a response to stress are common. 'Illness as theatre' often occurs, playing out the emotional story in the symptoms. Life not being sweet enough results in diabetes and extreme blood sugar swings, bitterness and disappointment in gallstones and so on. Another person may easily become entrapped in the saga as the 'care-giver' or, if it is projected, as the identified patient. The solar plexus is the point of digestion on all levels. It is where you assimilate, whether it be nourishment in the form of food, or an idea or an emotion. It is also where you can take on energy and emotions from outside yourself, especially when the chakra is stuck open. This chakra can have a powerful effect on your ability to assert yourself. The solar plexus represents radiant self-confidence and self-esteem – and your ability to laugh at yourself and the world. When functioning well it acts as a point of equilibrium between your present soul purpose and your past karma so that previous learning is applied wisely. You will have emotional stability and be able to express your feelings clearly. Linked to the intuition, the solar plexus chakra is also the seat of 'gut instincts' and bodily knowing. Blocked or blown, it can lead to taking on other people's feelings and problems, or to being overwhelmed by your own emotions. It affects energy assimilation and utilisation, and concentration. Emotional 'hooks' from other people can be found here.

Physiology: Adrenals, digestive system, liver, lymphatic system, metabolism, muscles, pancreas, skin, small intestine, stomach, eyesight.

Sense: Intuitive gut feelings, vision, self-awareness.

Positive quality: Empathic intuition.

Negative quality: Emotionally needy.

Overactive/blown/spin too fast: When this chakra is too open other people can all too easily draw on your energy and deplete you. Their emotions will rush into your subtle and physical bodies, overwhelming you with their feelings so that you lose track of your own. Your boundaries are diffuse. It is difficult to know where you end and someone else begins. You may receive 'wish-based' intuitions through your solar plexus as you unconsciously read other people's emotions. Equally, your own emotions will spill out, dumping on to everyone around you. You will feel hypersensitive and vulnerable, and have a tendency to wallow in ineffectual sympathy with others. It can lead you to endlessly try to fix in other people what you would be better attending to in yourself. You may be prey to wild intuitions, premonitions of doom and a paranoid suspicion that the whole world is out to get you. A blown solar plexus means you take on impressions from the external environment easily and these become attached and internalised.

Underactive/blocked/spin too slow: When this chakra is blocked you will be unable to share empathy or your own feelings with others – although you may still be overwhelmed by theirs. There will be a sense of inferiority and a tendency to cling too tightly or to push other people away. Intimacy and sharing is impossible when this chakra is blocked.

Typical dis-eases are emotional and demanding: Stomach ulcers, ME, 'fight or flight' adrenaline imbalances, SAD (seasonal affective disorder), insomnia and chronic anxiety, digestive problems and malabsorption, gallstones, pancreatic failure, liver problems, eczema and other skin conditions, eating disorders and phobias, multiple sclerosis.

Attachments: People with whom you have had an emotional entanglement in the past, whenever that may have been. Ancestral spirits, relatives, needy people. Invasion and energy leeching take place through this chakra, but your own outworn feelings and emotions can become attached here too and appear as external influences. External emotions, impressions and events can also leave their imprint.

The Heart Chakra (Anahata)
The sphere of unconditional love and nurturing
Location: Centre of chest, towards base of breastbone.

The Sanskrit name for this chakra means 'unstruck' or a 'sound that is made without two things striking'. The heart chakra is the core of your being: where the physical and the spiritual energies fuse and unconditional love thrives and is shared with others. It is the site of the bonds you make with other people, your relationships, and your interaction with the wider worlds around you. Unlimited, it is connected to 'All that Is'. When your heart chakra is open, you 'live from your heart' feeling safe and, therefore, compassionate. This is the basis of altruism, generosity and kindness – and respect for others. There is no judgement in an open heart chakra. Cooperation rather than competition flourishes. But your heart chakra is also the site of unselfish self-love. If you cannot love and accept yourself, then you cannot love others or receive their love. Self-love helps you to rise above egotism and asserts your self-worth. If your heart chakra is blocked, love cannot flourish, feelings such as jealousy are common and there is enormous resistance to change. When the heart is open and balanced, you trust yourself and your actions spontaneously arise from your heart not the head. Perceiving yourself as being loved, you will act out of compassion, giving love in return and sharing your resources. An open heart knows there will always be enough. It nurtures and shares – although it knows how to say 'no' and to keep appropriate bound-aries. This chakra is a connection centre that integrates the whole line of chakras along the spine. It helps you to realize that you are part of a much larger picture and opens the way to higher knowledge.

Physiology: Chest, circulation, heart, lungs, shoulders, thymus, respiratory system.

Sense: Touch, acceptance, perception of being loved.

Positive quality: Compassion and peaceful harmony.

Negative quality: Possessiveness.

Higher chakra connections: Higher heart and heart seed.

Overactive/blown/spin too fast: When this chakra is blown you are ruled by your emotions, reacting rather than responding. Happiness, sadness, anger, grief, neediness are overwhelming. Feelings and emotions are not processed and may be projected out to the world and perceived in the actions of others. This chakra has a strong connection to the past life chakras and previous life heartache may make itself felt, leading to a lack of trust. This chakra is vulnerable and can easily become codependent, needy and manipulative – and conditional. Your love will be based on 'I will only love you if...' and yet you will most probably be a people pleaser at the same time. 'Too much love' is common, indiscriminately pouring out sickly sweet love to cover self-perceived feelings of inadequacy, lack of self-worth and wanting – no matter how subconsciously – to make reparation for the past. This is the person who serves in order to be perceived as being a good person. But in relationships you will always be the giver, not the receiver. Balance will be lacking. You cover up or apologise for others, and constantly forgive, hanging on at all costs to a relationship that will most certainly not be for the highest good.

Underactive/blocked/spin too slow: Intimacy is a huge challenge when this chakra is closed off. With this chakra blocked you will feel undervalued and misunderstood. Emotions such as grief, anger, hatred, greed, envy and guilt are held on to, even nurtured. Feelings of inferiority, a sense of being unlovable and unloved, leads to a fear of rejection and a desperate desire not to be alone, but those very feelings push other people away. Or, you push them away before they can leave you. Equally you may settle for abusive or collusive relationships in order to satisfy the need not to be alone. The challenge is to overcome the fear that 'there will never be enough love'. This chakra holds on to past life pain and heartbreak. When blocked, it results in an inability to forgive yourself or those who have hurt you – and you have a hard time trusting people because your experiences 'confirm' that what you fear is true will come about, again and again. It is a self-fulfilling prophecy. You will probably set very high standards for yourself – and others – setting up a self-perpetuating loop whereby you are too hard on yourself, feel a failure and therefore experience both guilt and self-hatred. Energy from a blocked heart chakra can be subverted to the spleen, where it is experienced as anger attacking seemingly from outside. It may also be bounced back into the base and sacral chakra leading to sexual obsession.

Typical dis-eases are psychosomatic and reactive:

Heart attacks, angina, chest infections, asthma, frozen shoulder, ulcers, persistent cough, wheeziness, pneumonia, high cholesterol, mastitis, breast cysts, pancreatic problems.

Attachments: Family and ancestors, previous partners, authority or beloved figures, the needy and the desperate.

The Throat Chakra (Vishuddha)
The sphere of communication
Location: The centre of your throat.

The name of this chakra in Sanskrit means 'pure'. This chakra is all about communication and it can affect how valued and nurtured you feel. It is where you express yourself, including strongly felt feelings and emotions that come from the heart or solar plexus chakra as well as thoughts. If it is blocked and there is no outlet for these feelings and thoughts, it can lead to psychosomatic dis-ease. It can also lead to speaking what you think others wish to hear rather than being honest and sharing your heartfelt truth. You may feel that you have no right to express an opinion. If the chakra is functioning well you will freely express those opinions and be prepared to enter into debate about them and compromise or adjust with ease when appropriate. But you will also be able to stick to your principles when necessary. This chakra has a surprising amount to do with willpower and the choices that arise in life. It mediates our contact with the external world.

Physiology: Ears, nose, respiratory and nervous systems, sinuses, skin, throat, thyroid, parathyroid, tongue, tonsils, speech and body language, metabolism.

Sense: Hearing, expression and receiving.

Positive quality: Truthful self-expression. Available for communication.

Negative quality: Mendacity and evasiveness. Unavailable for communication.

Overactive/blown/spin too fast: A blown throat chakra creates a chatterbox who speaks unthinkingly, often to block out unacceptable feelings rising up from the solar plexus. Opinions, thoughts and feelings are blurted out indiscriminately. Or, it creates a control-freak who needs to be in charge and uses words to control how others think and feel, blocking out their emotions. Paradoxically, you may be too accepting of other people's views, lacking the capacity to reason things out for yourself. Energy may pour back down to the heart chakra, creating a tendency to be over-loving and overcompensating. The world may be experienced as uncaring because it cannot be communicated with – everything is going out, not being taken in and assimilated.

Underactive/blocked/spin too slow: If this chakra is blocked, your thoughts and feelings cannot be verbalized. Your truth cannot be expressed. You will not be able to stand up for yourself and may well be bullied. You may suffer from extreme shyness or believe that other people will not value, or will reject, what you have to say. You were probably told as a child that children should be seen and not heard. There will be a great fear of being judged and being unable to verbally defend or justify yourself. This chakra is also linked to listening and other people's opinions can cause you difficulties because you cannot allow yourself to perceive the truth of what they are saying. Nor engage in debate with them and put across your own point of view. The world may be experienced as hostile or pre-judging and so you reject it. A deficient or distorted throat chakra may also lead to egotism and judgementalism because other people's self-expression is feared, overruled or disregarded.

Typical dis-eases are active and block communication: Sore throat/quinsy, lump in throat, difficulty in swallowing, inflammation of trachea, sinus, constant colds and viral infections, tinnitus and ear infections, jaw pain and gum disease, tooth problems (related to root beliefs), thyroid imbalances, high blood pressure, ADHD, autism, speech impediment, psychosomatic diseases such as irritable bowel and metabolic dis-eases.

Attachments: Teachers, mentors, gurus, authority figures, thought forms. Problems can arise from your own unvoiced intuitions or thoughts which take on an external energetic form.

The Third Eye/Brow Chakra (Ajna)
The sphere of intuition and mental connection
Location: Above and between your eyebrows.

In Sanskrit the name of this chakra is 'command'. The brow chakra is where your inner sight meets your outer sight and bonds into intuitive insight. When this chakra is functioning well it connects to guides, mentors and higher beings. It helps you to see beyond consensual reality into what really *is*. It is the site of telepathy, clairvoyance and sensing unseen worlds and higher dimensions. But this metaphysical chakra also expresses the inner world and your spiritual connection. Imbalances here can create a sense of being bombarded by other people's thoughts, or being haunted by irrational intuitions that have no basis in truth. Controlling or coercing mental 'hooks' from other people may lock in and affect your thoughts. It can also have a surprising effect on mood. The brow chakra is closely linked to the pineal gland which monitors the amount of sunlight reaching you. In winter (in the northern hemisphere) when light levels are low, it slows down hormone production, conserving energy and lowering mood. In summer when light levels are high it boosts mood so this chakra acts as a mediator between your environment and your inner world. Opening your third eye can make your life smoother, but discretion is needed to ensure that it really is functioning at optimum and not accessing a level that is based on wishful thinking and illusion. If you develop a headache or migraine (common when this chakra is first opening up) during psychic work, open the chakra with Apophyllite or close it down with Flint until you can adjust your energies appropriately.

Physiology: Brain, ears, eyes, neurological and endocrine systems, pineal and pituitary glands, hypothalamus, production of serotonin and melatonin, temperature control, scalp, sinuses.

Sense: ESP, intuitive awareness.

Positive quality: Intuitive insight.

Negative quality: Delusion and illusion.

Overactive/blown/spin too fast: An overactive third eye can create a tendency to live in an escapist fantasy world, with a distorted view of reality. This is the overactive imagination going full steam ahead without constraint. Such rapid thought patterns can lead to being spaced out, or to having a one-track mind. It can result in uncontrolled contact with other, apparent, dimensions of reality as there is no filtering or discrimination as to what is perceived psychically. Lucid dreaming and out-of-body experiences will be common but not necessarily beneficial. There will be a greater awareness of auras and chakras, and you will be able to connect easily to spirit guides but these may not be of the highest quality. A blown chakra may manifest as, or create contact with, dishonesty, evasiveness, impatience, pride, egotism, arrogance, and authoritarianism – often because you or the person communicating sincerely believes that they are not only seeing true but also further than others and are therefore wiser. At the extreme it can lead to paranoia and schizoid behaviour. When too open, this chakra leaves you vulnerable to manipulation from those on other realms who may not have the highest good in mind. You may also act in a way that is manipulative and overbearing, feeling it is your God-given right.

Underactive/blocked/spin too slow: A blocked third eye leads to a lack of vision. There may be unhealthy attachment to a belief system or a guru. Narrow-mindedness, fear and cynicism are some of the consequences of a blocked third eye. You may be forgetful, an obsessive worrier or constantly doubting. It leads to ultra-linear rational thought or to muddled thinking with no ability to integrate insight and intuition with the intellect. The viewpoint is narrow and imagination may be severely impaired, so there will be problems with visualization. Blockages often occur in this chakra from childhood if you have been discouraged from speaking about what you see – physically or metaphysically – or from following your own inner guidance. This quickly leads to self-doubt and a lack of trust in your intuition. When this occurs there is a fear of success and 'imposter syndrome' (fear of being found out as not being who or as capable as you purport to be) is common. *Typical dis-eases* are intuitive and metaphysical: Migraines, mental overwhelm, schizophrenia, cataracts, iritis and other eye problems, epilepsy, autism, spinal and neurological disorders, sinus and ear infections, high blood pressure, learning disabilities, memory loss. Nervous or hormonal disorders, hot or cold flushes and excessive perspiration, 'irritations' of all kinds, skin conditions such as psoriasis, eczema, impetigo, allergies, sinus problems, adenoid and ear disorders, lack of energy and/or sex drive.

Attachments: Teachers, gurus and authority figures, thought forms, ancestors or relatives, lost souls.

The Crown Chakra (Sahasrara)
The sphere of spiritual communication and awareness
Location: Top of the head.

In Sanskrit this is the 'thousand petalled lotus'. An exceedingly powerful energy vortex. The crown chakra is the place of spiritual, intellectual and intuitive *knowing* so that you understand what is around you on many levels. It connects to multidimensions and multiverses. When kundalini reaches the crown chakra it opens a transcendent knowing. This chakra is linked to the 'master gland', the pituitary, which regulates homeostasis throughout your body keeping the endocrine system functioning efficiently. If the crown chakra is blocked, endocrine disturbances occur. If the crown chakra is not functioning well it can lead to excess environmental sensitivity, and to delusions or dementia. When the crown chakra connection is disturbed you are disconnected from your spiritual self and from cosmic energies. Spiritual interference or possession may result, and metabolic or psychological imbalances are common. If it is functioning well you express yourself as a spiritual being and attain unity consciousness. Your soul purpose will be accessed and actualised, leading you to self-understanding. You will be certain of your pathway and in tune with the cycles of life. You will recognize the lessons you programmed in before birth and find the gift in their heart.

Physiology: Brain, central nervous system, hair, hypothalamus, pituitary gland, spine, subtle energy bodies, cerebellum, nervous motor control, posture and balance.

Sense: Empathy, universal consciousness.

Positive quality: Spiritually connected.

Negative quality: Spiritual arrogance.

Overactive/blown/spin too fast: When this chakra is blown it leads to an overly imaginative, unfocused, spaced out and frustrated soul who is arrogant and uses power to control others. A blown crown is prey to illusions, undue influence and false communications. Obsession and openness to spiritual interference or possession can result. Attempting to control others is common as is 'false guru' syndrome. Energy can rush back down to the sexual chakras causing a psychotic breakdown or obsessive sexual expression.

Underactive/blocked/spin too slow: There can be no spiritual connection when this chakra is blocked. No interaction with your own higher self either, leading to feeling like an outsider or imposter. You will be indecisive, suffering from chronic exhaustion or excess frustration as you never seem to be getting anywhere in your spiritual search. You will have a blocked sense of power, leading to negative egotism. When this chakra is blocked it attracts put-downs and subtle attacks from other people – or from yourself as a self-defence mechanism.

Typical dis-eases arise out of disconnection and feelings of isolation: Metabolic syndrome, hypertension, 'unwellness' with no known cause, lethargy, nervous system disturbances, electromagnetic and environmental sensitivity, depression, dementia, ME, Parkinson's disease, insomnia or excessive sleepiness, 'biological clock' disturbances such as jet lag and seasonal affective disorder (SAD), impaired coordination, headaches, migraine, anxiety, depression, multiple personality disorder, mental breakdown.

Attachments: Spiritual entities, lost souls, mentors, gurus and 'alien intelligences'.

Exploring the Lesser Known Chakras

Our ability to grasp, to build, and to make our thoughts real lies inside this complex of bones, nerves, and vessels... The hand is a signature for who we are and what we can attain.
– Neil Shubin, *Your Inner Fish: A Journey into the 3.5 Billion Year History of the Human Body*

In addition to the seven well-known chakras, there are many so called minor chakras. I prefer to call these the lesser known as they can be powerful energy conduits and transformers. Activating the lesser known chakras will assist you in clearing anything that may be blocking your spiritual evolution and will help you to ground the higher dimension energies into everyday reality so that they actualise rather than remain in potential. Opening your palm chakras makes it much easier to feel or sense blockages and how energy is moving. It also enables you to receive energy. Anchoring yourself to the planet through your knee chakras brings the energy from the Earth up into your body and facilitates discharging negative or excess energy through the earth star as well. The spleen chakra gives you protection and the dantien power. The higher heart boosts your physical and psychic immune systems. Clearing the past life chakras means that you can move forward with no baggage, freed from the karmic deficits that would prevent you from stepping into a new frequency. It also facilitates drawing on your karmic wisdom, the fruit of all your previous lives wherever they took place.

The Palm Chakras
The sphere of energy manifestation, transmutation and utilisation
Location: The palms of your hands.

Hands are powerful sensors, part of a continual process of receiving and giving out. They assist you to interact with the world on an energetic level. The manifestation and healing chakras in the palm of your hand are what you use to *sense* energies. If you rub your hands together briskly and bring them together with fingers steepled and palms almost touching, these chakras tingle and pulsate. It will feel as though there is a ball of energy between your palms. The palm chakras are both receptive: receiving and sensing energy, and expressive: radiating and channelling it. So, they are intimately connected with your ability to receive and to generate, manifest and *actualise*. Fully functioning palm chakras help you to receive energy from the universe – or from crystals – and channel this into your energy field through the chakras. But they also project energy. This is where you experience expanded awareness and increased creativity in the physical and subtle energy worlds. The complex chakras are sited in the centre of your palms but the energy radiates up to your fingertips and as far as your elbows, possibly higher up the arms into the head and chest. Most people find that one hand is receptive and the other gives out energy. This varies according to whether you are left or right handed and with how your own energy field functions. Experiment to find which is right for you (see below). Always open your palm chakras before handling crystals and assessing the energy flow in the chakras and subtle bodies.

Physiology: Nerves, tendons, ganglions, skin, hands, fingers, nails.

Sense: Touch.

Positive quality: Manifestation, creativity, confidence. The palm chakra has the ability to facilitate transmutation of energy in addition to giving and receiving. When the chakra is functioning at optimum, you are able to receive in equal measure to giving. You will be receptive to love, compliments, advice and assistance but not be overly swayed by them. You will also channel unconditional love out to the world, particularly through what you create with your hands.

Negative quality: Grasping greed, numbness. Closed off and withdrawn from society, antisocial but paradoxically needy without knowing the reason why.

Connective correspondence: All the chakras but

especially the base and solar plexus.

Overactive/blown/spin too fast: Energy whirls out from the hands. You may constantly try to assist others but in an over-the-top, extreme way. Blown chakra hands are clumsy, easily breaking things, and may be physically abusive. They may form an outlet for anger, aggression or blocked assertive energy that is locked in the sacral chakra or solar plexus. Signs of a blown palm chakra include sweaty palms, hand wringing, itchy hands, hand rashes, peeling skin. There is a need to touch everything and an inability to let go. At the extreme this can become kleptomania.

Underactive/blocked/spin too slow: A blocked palm chakra results in a lack of creativity and the inability to express yourself artistically. Extreme touchiness is common. There is an inability to receive, including a refusal to ask for help or accept it when offered. Lack of connection with the world and with other people results in antisocial behaviour. At the extreme this becomes psychopathic or sociopathic. Unsociability includes refusing to share or to assist others in times of need. Nail or finger biting is common.

Typical dis-eases: Arthritis, brittle nails, carpal tunnel, Dupuytren's contracture, eczema, plantar fasciitis, psoriasis, rashes, allergies, shin splints, gut-disturbances, repetitive strain injury.

Attachments: Energy drawn from anyone you've shaken hands with or touched in any way; also negative energy from objects or the environment.

Activating your palm chakras

If you work frequently with crystals or are engaged in any kind of touch or healing, you will probably find that your palm chakras are already open. If not, however, it is easy to activate these.

- Concentrate on your hands and state your intention of opening the palm chakras.
- Rapidly open and close your fingers, making a fist five or six times.
- Concentrate your attention into your right hand palm and then your left. (If you are left handed reverse the process.) Picture them opening like petals. The centres become hot and energized.
- Bring your cupped hands together. Stop as soon as you feel the energy of the two chakras meeting. Move your hands backwards and forwards a little until you know exactly how far the energy extends.
- With a little practice you'll be able to open the chakras simply by putting your attention there.

Establishing receptivity and energy radiation

- Place a crystal point across your hand. Feel the energies radiating into your palm. Change hands and note which palm chakra seems to best receive the energy.
- Turn the point towards your arm and then towards your fingers. Be aware of the direction of the energy flow. (Points channel energy in the

direction they face.)

- Practise sensing the energy flow from the chakra along your arms by running your hand slowly up your arm. Does it feel hot, cold, buzzy, still? Balanced and harmonious or jangly or depleted? Then change hands to see which senses the energy most strongly. This will be the hand you use to feel blockages and energy flow.
- Then practise sending energy into your chakras, holding your hand over each one in turn – visualize it moving from your palm into the chakra. Change hands and see which hand radiates energy most strongly. This will be the hand you use to remove blockages and harmonize energy flow.

The Knee Chakras

The sphere of flexibility, balance and willpower

Location: Behind and through the knees, like a flat disc on which the body rests.

When working well the knee chakras ensure you are flexible and able to adapt to changing circumstances. Literally able to 'go with the flow' and yet having perseverance when required. You are able to use your willpower to manifest a desired outcome rather than to insist on it. All the major energy meridians of the body pass through the knees as well as the longest nerve in the body, the sciatic. These chakras ensure that you have the ability to nurture and support yourself and manifest what you need on a day-to-day basis. When the knee chakras are balanced, you can set realistic goals and outcomes, and let go when appropriate. You will also have humility and can offer service to others from an open heart. Not only can the knee chakras be blocked or too open, but they can also suffer a left-right imbalance so check out each chakra and harmonize them with appropriate crystals. Generally speaking (but check it out for yourself), the left knee represents the feminine, yin aspect, that is receptive, emotional and intuitive. It is connected to the intuitive right hemisphere of the brain. The right knee represents the male, yang, aspect that is factual, practical, managerial and outgoing. It is connected to the rational left side of the brain.

Physiology: Brain, kidneys, lumbar spine, heart, bladder and kidney meridians, sciatic nerve.

Sense: Balance.

Positive quality: The ability to move forward with confidence. Well grounded and practical. Basic needs are fulfilled with ease. Is naturally respected, does not demand it.

Negative quality: Hare-brained, inflexible, or servile. Fear of change, especially of death.

Connective chakra correspondence: The earth star, base, sacral and dantien.

Overactive/blown/spin too fast: When this chakra is blown, you will be overly impulsive and act before thinking, aggressively pushing through obstacles. You will be unable to negotiate or compromise. A blown knee chakra constantly meets problems with authority, authority figures and bureaucracy. There is a need to be in control. Arrogant superiority is common. This is the person who thinks he, or she, 'knows best', so demands subservience from others. Control-freakery is common as is jumping from the frying pan into the fire.

Underactive/blocked/spin too slow: Chronic fear and feelings of inferiority, and consequent subservience result from blocked knee chakras. Unhealthy dependent and controlling relationships including 'codependency', or difficulties in intimacy and closeness are common. You will be constantly challenged by others. Someone with blocked knee chakras experiences a lack of basic sustenance, materially and nutritionally. Needs are not met and so you are focused on what is lacking rather than what is there. The soul is not grounded into the earth plane, or practical everyday reality, and so feels empty.

Typical dis-eases: Frequent knee problems, arthritis, water on the knee, cartilage and joint problems, bladder problems, cold feet, Osgood-Schlatter disease, bursitis, osteoarthritis, poor leg circulation, sacroiliac pain, lumbar spine, cystitis, eating disorders, malabsorption of nutrients, kidney diseases.

Attachments: Those who want you to walk in their footsteps – ancestral spirits or past life personas that have a different agenda to your soul.

Anchoring the knee chakras

Balancing and opening the knee chakras helps you to ground and assimilate the energies and to maintain your connection to the Earth. Placing an appropriate crystal on each knee facilitates this.

- Sitting rather than standing, repeat the grounding root crystal visualization on page 34.
- When the grounding root is in place, place an appropriate knee chakra crystal on each knee – you may need different crystals for each knee according to how the individual chakras are functioning (dowse to check, see page 169).
- Feel how the energy locks into the grounding root pathways and helps them to flow.
- Leave the crystals in place for five to fifteen minutes. If appropriate, tape in place overnight.
- Repeat as often as necessary until the energy flows easily in both directions or as directed by the power of your mind.

The Dantien

The sphere of power

Location: Two fingerbreadths (3–5 cm) below the navel, rotating on top of the sacral.

The dantien is an energy vortex and storage vault rather than a chakra per se. A powerpoint, the dantien acts as a higher resonance of the sacral chakra. An adjunct to the sacral chakra and the point of balance for the physical body, the dantien is where Qi or prana, life force, is stored and your body earthed. Acting like a reservoir, this is your core energy source. It is a place of inner strength, stability and balance. This chakra is where you become centred around your inner core. When you are connected to your core, you not only have more physical energy as you are not affected by life's ups and downs, but you are also more emotionally stable and better able to resist stress. You are not easily thrown off balance. Nor are you open to manipulation by other people. When the dantien is full, you have inner resources to draw on. You are literally power-full. When it is functioning well you are energized and power-full, stable and well grounded. If the dantien is too open, you are labile, frenetic and energy is constantly drained.

Physiology: Autonomic nervous and energy-conduction systems, regulation of the internal organs and involuntary processes such as breathing and heartbeat. Sensory impulses to the brain.

Sense: Balance and positive self-assertion.

Positive quality: Powerful-ness.

Negative quality: Depletion and neediness.

Connective correspondence: Higher resonance of the sacral chakra.

Overactive/blown/spin too fast: If the dantien is too open, energy constantly drains out and chronic lethargy results. Many projects will be started but you will have no stamina or perseverance to complete them. You will also be easily pushed around or manipulated by other people, despite feeling that you are in control.

Underactive/blocked/spin too slow: Qi (life force) cannot circulate efficiently and is not replenished. The autoimmune system cannot function, with resultant disease. Ideas cannot be put into practice and creativity is blocked.

Typical dis-eases relate to physical function and energy utilisation: Nervous system dysfunctions, autoimmune diseases, cardiac problems, high blood pressure, orthostatic hypotension, palpitations, adrenal overload, chronic fatigue, ME, Raynaud's, Parkinson's, digestive problems, diabetes, light-headedness, powerlessness, feeling ill at ease in incarnation.

Attachments: Energy leeches, control freaks, disembodied spirits seeking energy to re-manifest or move on.

Charging up the dantien

Charging up your dantien makes an enormous amount of difference to how much energy you have available and how easily you cope with the ups and downs of life.

- Stand with your feet firmly on the floor and knees slightly flexed. Sit back on your pelvis so that you feel centred and balanced.
- Hold a Carnelian or other dantien activation crystal in both hands just below your navel.
- Be aware of the energy of the stone radiating into the dantien.
- Breathe deeply, pulling the breath down to the

dantien as you breathe in, and holding the energy in the dantien as you breathe out.

- The area under the crystal will become hot and energized.
- When you have finished, place your hands over the dantien to close the external portal to the energy vortex so that other people cannot draw on your energy. Be aware that you have an inner reservoir of power to call on which can be pulled up your spine to energize other chakras when needed or sent down to the base to recharge your creative juices and basic life force.
- Five minutes a day should be sufficient to fully charge up your dantien but if you need more energy at any time, keep your crystal in a pocket as close as possible to the dantien.

The Spleen Chakra

The sphere of self-protection and empowerment

Location: A hand's breadth below the left armpit extending down towards the waist, back and front.

This chakra should not be confused with the sacral chakra (sometimes erroneously called the spleen). When the chakra is wide open, other people can draw on your energy, leaving you depleted particularly at the immune and vitality levels. If you have a constant ache under your left armpit then the chakra is too open and a psychic vampire has hooked in to get their energy fix. If the chakra is balanced, energy can easily flow around your physical and subtle bodies and you are protected. When the chakra is blocked, emotional energy especially anger can become stuck there and this will also deplete you.

There is a corresponding chakra on the right side of the body, over the liver. If, having removed hooks from your spleen chakra, you get a pain under the right armpit this is the result of an energy vampire becoming frustrated at having the power source cut off. This can be easily be dealt with (see below). This closing of the energy portal cuts off energy vampires among the living as well as those who have passed over but not let go.

Physiology: Spleen, pancreas, lymphatic system and liver.

Sense: Safety and security.

Positive quality: Self-assertive and empowered.

Negative quality: Aggression and vampirisation.

Connective correspondence: Solar plexus and heart.

Overactive/blown/spin too fast: If this chakra is wide open then anyone can hook into your energy and deplete you. You will pick up other people's feelings, especially anger and irritation which can lead to physical pain. You will remain connected to anyone with whom you have had close contact. People can easily take advantage of you, manipulating and coercing you into self-destructive actions that are not for your highest good. Your body may well turn in to attack itself leading to autoimmune diseases. Uncontrollable anger is common when this chakra is blown as you unconsciously rebel against being subtly manipulated or vampirised.

Underactive/blocked/spin too slow: When this chakra is blocked you will feel rootless, purposeless, exhausted and manipulated, powerless. You may well have anger issues but find it difficult to express your anger. You may also suffer constant irritation, some of which goes back to unresolved past life issues. As with the blown chakra, your body may turn in to attack itself. Intimacy with others is impossible when this chakra is locked shut.

Typical dis-eases are those of depletion and lack: Lethargy, anaemia, low blood sugar, diabetes, pancreatitis, liver problems, autoimmune diseases.

Attachments: Psychic vampires, needy people, ex-partners, soul parts from previous incarnations/dimensions that have not been integrated and which may have a different soul purpose to your own.

Closing and protecting the spleen energy portal

Keeping your spleen chakra free from hooks should be a regular part of your spiritual and energetic house-keeping. This is quickly achieved with a crystal.

- Cleanse your spleen chakra by spiralling out a Quartz point, Flint, raw Charoite or Rainbow Mayanite to clear any hooks or energetic connections from the chakra, or use a Jasper or Sard tie-cutter.
- To protect the chakra after tie cutting, tape a

Tantalite, Green Aventurine, Green Fluorite or Jade crystal over the spleen chakra, or wear one on a long chain so that it reaches to the end of your breastbone level with the chakra.

- Picture a three-dimensional green pyramid extending down from your armpit to your waist, front and back to protect the spleen.
- If the area under your right armpit then begins to ache, tape a piece of Gaspeite, Tugtupite or Bloodstone over the site and leave in place for several days until the message is received that you will not be giving away any more of your energy. You can also picture a red three-dimensional pyramid protecting this area.

The Higher Heart (Thymus) Chakra
The sphere of well-being
Location: Over the thymus gland, between the heart and the throat.

This chakra governs the physical and psychic immune systems and how you protect yourself. It has a profound effect on well-being in general. It is the site of production of the T-cells that are responsible for fending off disease, and is highly susceptible to stress. This chakra is over the thymus gland, the first gland to develop in the uterus and, therefore, a core component of how your body functions *in utero*, what genetic potential gets switched on, and how much natural immunity you will have throughout life. Connected to ancestral DNA and to the past life patterning you carry in your body, if this chakra is blocked these will hold sway. Your physical body will reflect the blockages through a compromised immune system and consequent dis-eases. At the level of the psyche, if this chakra is not functioning well you will be emotionally needy and unable to express your feelings openly as it mediates and expresses a synthesis of the heart and throat. At a spiritual level, unconditional love and service cannot be offered if the chakra is blocked or blown. When it is functioning at optimum, it opens the compassionate heart.

Physiology: The psychic and physical immune systems, thymus gland, lymphatic system, elimination and purification organs.

Sense: Protection.

Positive quality: Well protected, unconditional love, forgiving, accepting, spiritually connected.

Negative quality: Paranoid, spiritually disconnected, grieving, needy, a psychic vampire.

Chakra connection: forms the three-chambered heart chakra with the heart and heart seed chakras.

Overactive/blown/spin too fast: When this chakra is wide open the immune system turns in on itself, destroying the body and its cells. There is no protection against toxins from outside, nor internal emotional toxicity.

Underactive/blocked/spin too slow: When this chakra is blocked the immune system cannot function at optimum. It allows bacteria and viruses to run riot through your system and negative ancestral DNA patterns to predominate.

Typical dis-eases reflect a blocked or disordered immune system: Autoimmune diseases, repeated viral and bacterial infections, coughs, colds, glandular fever, ME, MS, HIV/AIDS, arteriosclerosis, flushing of the chest and neck, tinnitus, epilepsy, vitiligo, psoriasis, alopecia, thyroid problems.

Attachments: Guides, gurus or masters, mentors. Mentors, masters and gurus open the higher heart chakra, and in so doing tie you to them and not all masters or gurus have clean energy or the best of intentions.

The Past life Chakras
The sphere of memory and hereditary issues
Location: Three fingers breadth behind your ears, and along the bony ridge to the base of the skull.

The past life chakras are where you store the memories of your previous lives, deeply ingrained soul programs, and emotional baggage from the past. They hold all the traumas, dramas, gifts and lessons you have learned over many lifetimes and may well be holding on to outdated soul intentions from previous lives. This elongated dual chakra links to the karmic blueprint which has the soul wounds, physical and emotional, from the past embedded in it. This can create psychosomatic dis-ease or actual physical disease which is carried through engrams or subtle memory traces. An engram is a mental image that records an experience containing pain, unconsciousness and a real or fancied threat to survival. An engram can be created in a past life and carried over to the present through the karmic blueprint. Activating these chakras can bring up many memories to be released but they can also help you to reconnect to soul gifts that you have developed in the past.

Physiology: The karmic blueprint and etheric bodies. Wounds, attitudes and dysfunction in these subtle bodies imprint on to the physical at a psychosomatic or genetic level. Psychological dis-eases impact on the mind and from there on to the body.

Sense: Memory and sense perception.

Positive quality: Self-directed.

Negative quality: Ruled by the past.

Higher chakra connection: Causal vortex.

Overactive/blown/spin too fast: When these chakras are wide open, there is no filter and no understanding of what is past and what is present. Past life experiences constantly impinge on the present to the extent that there may be emotional or psychiatric disturbances. Deep fear, paranoia and other manifestations are common. Emotional baggage and unfinished business constantly sabotage daily life. When the chakras are blown, you will feel unsafe and subconsciously overwhelmed by past life memories of trauma, violent death and fears. This leaves the way open for past life personas, soul fragments and thought forms to attach or re-manifest.

Underactive/blocked/spin too slow: Blockages here

mean that you are stuck in the past and cannot move forward. You may well be repeating your own past life patterns or recreating ancestral patterns that have passed down through your family. Considerable cleansing work may be needed to clear the imprints, memories and engrams from the past that are lodged here (see the Directory, past life issues page 301).

Typical dis-eases: Chronic illnesses, especially immune or endocrine deficiencies, genetic or physical malfunctions. Physical illnesses reflect previous life wounds, such as pain or stiffness in the particular part of the body that was injured. Psychosomatic illnesses that reflect deeply held attitudes and beliefs manifest as heart, liver or kidney problems or autoimmune diseases.

Attachments: Past life personas, soul fragments, thought forms from previous beliefs. This is a point where people from the past can attach and control you.

Opening the Personal Chakras and Integrating the Lesser Known

A simple crystal layout will cleanse and open the personal chakras so that the lesser known can then be integrated into the system.

Personal chakra cleanse, balance and recharge

- Place Smoky Quartz or other earth star crystal between and slightly below your feet. Picture light and energy radiating out from the crystal into the earth star for two or three minutes and be aware that the chakra is being cleansed and its spin regulated.
- Place Red Jasper or other base chakra crystal on the base chakra. Picture light and energy radiating out from the crystal into the base chakra as before.
- Place Orange Carnelian or other sacral chakra crystal on your sacral chakra, just below the navel; see the light and feel the cleansing process.
- Place Yellow Jasper or other solar plexus crystal on your solar plexus.

- Place Green Aventurine or other heart chakra crystal on your heart.
- Place Blue Lace Agate or other throat chakra crystal on your throat.
- Place Sodalite or other third eye chakra crystal on your brow.
- Place Amethyst or other crown chakra crystal on your crown.
- Breathe deeply taking the breath all the way down to your feet as you inhale, and then letting your attention come slowly up your body as you exhale until you reach your crown. Repeat several times.
- Remain still and relaxed, breathing deep down into your belly and counting to seven before you exhale. As you breathe in and hold, feel the energy of the crystals re-energizing the chakras and from there radiating out through your whole being.
- Now take your attention slowly from the soles of your feet up the midline of your body feeling how each chakra has become balanced and harmonized.
- When you feel ready, gather your crystals up, starting from the crown. As you reach the earth chakra, be aware of a grounding cord anchoring you to the Earth and into your physical body.
- Cleanse your stones thoroughly (see page 173).

Integrating the lesser known chakras

Once the personal chakras are up and running efficiently, introduce the lesser known chakras such as the knees and the dantien into the above layout, placing an appropriate crystal. When the lesser known chakras have been cleansed and activated, allow the energy to flow and be incorporated into the personal chakra alignment.

The Microcosmic Crystal Orbit

Once all the chakras have been aligned, it is possible to circulate Qi, otherwise known as prana or life force, through the chakras so that it energizes the physical and subtle energy bodies. Any excess can be stored in the dantien until required. Qi is not the same as kundalini. It is a life force energy but not at such a concentrated, high vibrational resonance as kundalini, being more earthy in nature. Therefore, rather than uplifting you spiritually, this effervescent force uplifts your physical vibrations and infuses them with vitality and verve. It is a power source that the physical body can utilise at any time for well-being, enthusiasm and good health. The microcosmic orbit comes from the Qigong tradition and the addition of a crystal infuses it with even more dynamic potential.

The microcosmic orbit

You will need a Qi-enhancing base chakra or dantien crystal such as Red or Poppy Jasper, Eye of the Storm, Red Amethyst or Carnelian (see the Directory page 309).

- Hold your Qi crystal in your hands and let your arms drop as low as possible so that the crystal sits between the base and sacral chakras.
- Feel the base of your spine light up as the Qi stirs. Your base chakra will fire up.
- Breathe deep down into your belly and visualize that energy moving up the back of your spine from the base into the sacral chakra and the dantien. As it goes it enlivens and invigorates the organs, meridians and glands associated with each chakra so that the energy passes into your physical and subtle energy bodies.
- Feel the energy moving on up through your solar plexus and the three-chambered heart, energizing as it goes.
- Sense the energy moving up through your throat chakra and into the back of your skull. Here it energizes the base of the alta major and then moves over the back of your head to the crown chakra at the top.
- At the crown chakra the Qi begins its journey back down the chakras at the front of the body. It is helpful to put the tip of your tongue to the roof of your mouth to facilitate the energy moving through the mouth. When it has passed down the front of your body and reaches the dantien it is stored there until needed again.
- Continue to circulate Qi for five or ten minutes until the dantien feels fully activated and your

whole body is invigorated.

Note: If you begin to feel light-headed, floaty and ungrounded at any time during this exercise place a Flint, Hematite, Boji Stone or Smoky Quartz at your feet and put your grounding cord in place (see page 34). If kundalini begins to move, use Anandalite or Serpentine to control the flow moving it slowly upwards to the crown and down again to the base and dantien. You will recognize the difference between Qi and kundalini by the wild fieriness of the latter.

Expanding Awareness: The Higher Vibrational, Soul Level, Chakras

Familiarising yourself with additional chakras greatly enhances your crystal experience. These chakras are coming on line to facilitate the assimilation of higher dimensional energy but you may find that you have been using them for some time without necessarily being aware of it... But, if not, you can soon have these powerful energy points working for you.
– Judy Hall, *Crystal Bible 3*

Higher vibrational chakras that have previously been lying dormant are coming on line as energy shifts occur and consciousness is raised. These chakras assist in assimilating the changing frequencies, connecting to higher beings and exploring other dimensions. If you are a beginner, higher chakra activation is best done slowly one chakra at a time. Ensure that a chakra is functioning well before you move on to the next one. But, if you have been raising your vibrations already, these chakras may have opened spontaneously and may need regulating and rebalancing, which is where crystals can assist.

The higher crown chakras include the soul star and the stellar gateway but there are many more chakras above the head, going way up through exceedingly high vibrations, multidimensions and multiverses. New stones will undoubtedly continue to appear over the next few years as these chakras open up. It is essential to have fully grounded and integrated all the chakras below, up to and including the stellar gateway before these can be fully utilised, and it is beyond the scope of this book to include these additional chakras at this time. There is a point where the higher chakras become a dimension in themselves rather than an energy vortex that is more or less restricted to a four-dimensional realm.

The Gaia Gateway Chakra
The sphere of anchoring Light

Location: About arm's length beneath your feet, below the earth star. (Note: in other systems this chakra is perceived as just above and to the side of your navel but it serves the same function.)

A higher resonance of the earth star, this chakra anchors high frequency light into the physical body and the body of the Earth. Without this chakra high vibrational energy cannot be assimilated and grounded. It adjusts your electromagnetic frequency so that it remains in harmonic resonance with that of the planet *and* facilitates an uplift in your own personal resonance. It, together with the stellar gateway, allows kundalini energy to travel up the spine, into the higher chakras over the head, and then to cascade down through the subtle energy bodies into the Gaia gateway. The energy then travels back up to the dantien where it can be stored until needed, or moves out in the cells and intercellular spaces of the physical and subtle bodies. This chakra connects you to the soul and spirit of the planet, Gaia, and to Mother Earth herself. When your Gaia gateway is open and functioning at optimum, you are aware of being a part of a sacred whole, part of the energy system of the Earth and, at the same time, All That Is. When balanced and open, this chakra helps you to protect yourself from entity attachment and lower energies. By holding you gently in incarnation and in contact with the planet, it mitigates the more extreme symptoms of ascension and kundalini rise.

Physiology: Subtle energy bodies beyond the physical, linking into the Earth's subtle bodies and meridian system.

Sense: At-one-ness.

Positive quality: The soul is fully grounded within the human and earthy spheres and aware of the divine.

Negative quality: Disconnected or oversensitive.

Connective correspondence: Stellar gateway.

Overactive/blown/spin too fast: When this chakra is blown it leads to extreme sensitivity to Earth changes and to geopathic and electromagnetic stress. Being in incarnation, and especially being in a physical body, is challenging and there is no ability to remain stable during periods of energetic uplift.

Underactive/blocked/spin too slow: When this chakra is blocked there is an inability to ground and connect with higher energies. Disconnection from the Earth as a sacred, living being may lead to greed and over-utilisation of the planet's resources and consequent disregard for others who share the planet.

Typical diseases are beyond the scope of the physical although inability to ground kundalini and higher consciousness can lead to many and varied symptoms (see Kundalini page 152).

The Soma Chakra
The sphere of soul-body connection

Location: Above the third eye, at the mid hairline. Known in Sanskrit as 'the healing nectar chakra' this is where the twin forces of Shiva, the divine, and Shakti, kundalini power, meet. It can also be seen with a psychic eye as the place where the masculine and feminine currents of the body entwine and meld with the divine creating a point of oneness and non-duality. It has traditionally been regarded as a sphere of rejuvenation and immortality. Being the location where the etheric and lightbodies are attached to the physical, it is the anchor for the 'silver cord' that holds the subtle energy bodies in contact with the physical during journeying and out-of-body experiences. A higher resonance of the third eye, when activated the soma chakra opens metaphysical awareness and visionary ability. The chakra also links to the angelic realms and spirit guides. It has to do with perception of the cycles of time and awareness of the workings of synchronicity. When this chakra is functioning well it gives you the mental clarity necessary to achieve en-lighten-ment and promotes lucid dreaming. It unites the pituitary gland which governs physical function with the pineal, transcendent spiritual awareness. However, when this chakra is blown it is all too easy for discarnate spirits to attach or for you to be subject to involuntary out-of-body experiences that may literally blow your mind.

Physiology: The whole body including the etheric and lightbodies and the subtle energy systems, the pineal and pituitary glands.

Sense: Connection.

Positive quality: Spiritually aware and fully conscious.

Negative quality: Disconnected and cut off from spiritual nourishment.

Connective correspondence: Third eye, throat and soul star chakras.

Overactive/blown/spin too fast: When this chakra is blown it is difficult for the subtle bodies to remain anchored in the physical realm. Spontaneous out-of-body experiences, wild delusions, and a frenetic or manic energy result. A person with a blown soma chakra may appear to be deeply spiritual, channelling higher dimensional energies, but it is doubtful if the contact is genuinely evolved, and delusions are common.

Underactive/blocked/spin too slow: When this chakra

is blocked 'the nectar of healing' cannot flow. Fluidity is lost and spirituality dries up. Physically it results in accelerated ageing, dryness of skin and dehydration. At a psychic level, the subtle bodies cannot leave the physical realm to be recharged by spiritual forces. The intuition cannot function and the soul cannot go home.

Typical dis-eases are autistic and disconnected or dyspraxic and may include Down's Syndrome, autism and ADHD, chronic fatigue, delusional states. Blockages may also manifest as sinus or eye problems, migraine headaches, stress headaches, digestive difficulties.

Attachments: 'Lost souls', walk-ins, gurus.

The Soul Star
The sphere of ultimate soul awareness

Location: About a foot above your head.

An interface for relationship with the universe and beyond, the soul star is a bridge between spirit and matter. This chakra adjusts extremely high spiritual frequencies so they can be integrated into matter. When assimilated by the physical body, they can be expressed here on Earth. When not functioning at optimum, this chakra may lead to spiritual arrogance, soul fragmentation or a messiah-complex. It is the person who rescues and enslaves others rather than empowers them. It can also be the site of spirit attachment, ET invasion, or overwhelm by ancestral spirits. When functioning at optimum there is true humility, with a connection to overall soul intention and an objective perspective on the past that leads to spiritual illumination. This chakra also holds the collective karma of humankind and the history of the evolution of the cosmos.

Physiology: The subtle bodies and their effect on the psyche.

Positive qualities: Attuned to the highest vibrations. True humility.

Negative qualities: Spiritual arrogance and interference, soul fragmentation.

Chakra correspondence: Earth star, causal vortex, stellar gateway.

Overactive/blown/spin too fast: When this chakra is spinning out of control it leads to spiritual arrogance or a messiah complex, a feeling of knowing all the answers and a compulsion to compel others to follow what is taught. No debate or dissension is allowed. Alternatively, and alternately, it can lead to feelings of spiritual isolation and desolation as soul connection is lost. When there is no control over this chakra it may lead to soul fragmentation or spirit attachment, ET invasion, or overwhelm by ancestral spirits and their unfulfilled desires.

Underactive/blocked/spin too slow: If this chakra is blocked there is little or no awareness of being an eternal spirit who happens to be in physical incarnation at the present time, and equally no connection to higher beings or to your own higher energies. The viewpoint is consequentially narrow, materialistic and greedy or needy. You may well feel that you have no right to exist at all and constantly apologise for yourself. You may also feel that you are the cause of other people's problems and try to make reparation or force a resolution on their behalf. Unresolved past life issues and previous soul imperatives may well be ruling your life.

Typical dis-eases are psychological and psychiatric: Schizophrenia, paranoia, bipolar disorder.

Attachments: Ancestral spirits, ETs, 'lost souls', soul parts that are not in incarnation and which may have their own agenda.

The Stellar Gateway
The cosmic doorway to other worlds

Location: Above the Soul Star.

The stellar gateway is a dimensional portal rather than a physical site. It is a point of connection to the divine and to the multiverses surrounding us: where the soul can make a connection to its own higher self, other realms, higher dimensions and All That Is. When this chakra is imbalanced the soul will be fragmented, disintegrated, unable to function in the everyday world. The disconnected soul results in a 'space cadet' who is open to cosmic disinformation as it is the lower astral plane rather than higher dimensions with which connection will be made. When functioning optimally, two-way communication with higher dimensional beings is possible and spiritual illumination results.

Physiology: Beyond the physical.

Positive quality: Soul communication.

Negative quality: Disinformation.

Connective correspondence: Gaia gateway.

Overactive/blown/spin too fast: A blown stellar gateway leaves you open to illusions, and a source of cosmic disinformation that leads to delusion, deception and disintegration leaving you unable to function in the everyday world.

Underactive/blocked/spin too slow: A blocked stellar gateway means you are unable to connect to the soul or higher dimensions. There is a feeling that the material realm is all that there is, and so spiritual qualities such as empathy and compassion are lacking and ego runs rife.

Typical dis-eases are beyond the physical and arise out of spiritual and soul disconnection.

Attachments: So-called enlightened beings that are anything but.

The Alta Major (Ascension) Chakra
The sphere of expanding awareness

Location: Inside the skull.

Also known as the 'ascension chakra', the alta major is a major factor in accelerating and expanding consciousness. An anchor for the multidimensional lightbody, it unites metaphysical sight and intuitive insight. When balanced, the alta major gives the ability to see the bigger picture. All the pieces of the jigsaw puzzle of life fit in place. It enhances intuitive ideas and makes them more solid, tangible and achievable. This chakra holds valuable information about our ancestral past and the ingrained patterns that govern human life and awareness. It, in conjunction with the causal vortex and past life chakras, contains your past life karma and the contractual agreements you made with your Higher Self and others before incarnating in this lifetime. Activating it enables you to read your soul's plan. Its link to the throat chakra facilitates expression of information from higher dimensions. Opening this chakra allows you to instinctively know your spiritual purpose. Many of the new high vibration crystals activate the alta major and facilitate multidimensional awareness, the ability to operate in several dimensions at once. Reputedly the alta major chakra has been imprinted with 'divine codes' that, when activated, will allow cosmic evolution to fully manifest on Earth. If the alta major is functioning well your subtle endocrine system harmonizes the subtle bodies with the physical. You will have a strong sense of direction in life and a well-functioning immune system.

The chakra creates a complex, merkaba-like geometric shape within the skull that stretches from the base of the skull to the crown connecting the past life and soma chakras, hippocampus, hypothalamus, pineal and pituitary glands with the third eye, soma and higher crown chakras. Known since ancient times as 'the third eye' and more recently as 'the seat of the soul', the pineal gland works in conjunction with the subtle energy structure of the alta major. Along with the hypothalamus it is the body's light meter and body clock regulator, sending out physiological-timing hormones in response to the amount of light reaching the eyes. But in addition, the pineal contains crystalline 'brain sand', hydroxyapatite (found in Apatite, Fluorapatite and other crystals), which holds crystalline information. This metaphysical gland acts as a multidimensional energy structure into which higher vibrational energies can anchor. It has been postulated that the pineal secretes DMT, often called the 'spirit molecule'. A natural psychedelic, DMT is involved in out-of-body, near-death and other exceptional human experiences that take the soul into multidimensions and expanded vision. So, when the alta major is activated in conjunction with the pineal gland and the third eye chakra, metaphysical abilities, especially telepathy and far sight, function with greater clarity (see The Crystal Palace page 145 and my *Book of Psychic Development*).

The activation point for this chakra is connected to the hypothalamus, deep inside the brain. A 'puppet master', the hypothalamus is responsible for synchronizing the body's biological clock by sending information to the pineal and pituitary, and for coordinating the interface between the body, mind and environment. Its primary function is homeostasis, maintaining and balancing the body's status quo throughout the whole organism. The hormones it produces are responsible for body temperature, thirst, hunger, sleep, circadian rhythm, moods, sex drive, blood pressure, body weight and growth. So the alta major chakra governs the behavioural, autonomic, and endocrine functions that keep the body in harmony with external factors. It could be said to help you become one with the universe – one of the products of kundalini activation.

The alta major also encompasses the hippocampus, a major source of spatial orientation that enables you to navigate your way through life. It is involved in memory forming, organizing, and storing including your emotional responses. Acting as a memory indexer, it sends memories to long-term storage and retrieves them when necessary. Bringing all these glands into synchronized functioning and raising their frequency with an influx of kundalini within a balanced alta major vastly improves well-being and expands consciousness – although an overloading produces many of the major side effects of kundalini.

Physiology: The subtle and physical endocrine systems including the hippocampus, hypothalamus, pineal and pituitary glands; brain function, the cerebellum and voluntary muscle movements, the medulla oblongata controlling breathing, heart rate and blood pressure; hormonal balance, occipital area and the optic nerve, throat, spine, sleeping patterns.

Senses: All.

Positive quality: This chakra creates a direct pathway between your conscious, subconscious and intuitive minds and the higher universal mind. Opening it allows you to instinctively know your spiritual purpose. Its link to the throat chakra facilitates expression of information from higher dimensions.

Negative quality: Disorientation and discombobulation.

Chakra connection: Throat, third eye, past life, causal vortex, crown.

Overactive/blown/spin too fast: When this chakra is blown memories flood in too fast to process, and overwhelm the psyche. You will feel disorientated, open to paranoid delusions – which will feel like reality – and will be acutely attuned to subtle disturbances in the environment around you. You may feel like you've been taken over by something outside yourself. The physiology of the physical body will be out of kilter with disturbances created by overproduction of hormones.

Underactive/blocked/spin too slow: When this chakra is blocked memories of the past will be clung to and will govern behaviour. Inner sight cannot open and new information cannot be processed. The physiology of the body will be out of kilter with disturbances caused by underproduction of hormones.

Typical diseases are ancestral, karmic or those of disorientation: Metabolic dysfunction, eye problems, floaters, cataracts, migraine, headaches, memory loss, Alzheimer's or dementia and feelings of confusion, physical depression, 'dizziness' or 'floatiness', loss of sense of purpose and spiritual depression, fear, terror, adrenaline rush.

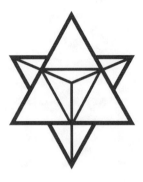

Merkaba shape

The Causal Vortex (Galactic) Chakra
The record of the soul's journey

Location: 3–4 inches above and behind the head (dowse for its exact placement).

Acting rather like a universal and cosmic worldwide web, the causal vortex accesses the Akashic Records especially that of your own soul. It assists in assessing how far you have travelled on your spiritual journey and how well you are doing with your karmic lessons. When this chakra is operational, the spiritual will is activated, guided by the Higher Self and the universal mind. It receives wisdom and guidance from spiritual mentors and higher dimensional beings. Accessing this chakra illuminates the things you have chosen to experience in a given physical life and what lessons you are trying to learn. It is also a repository for ancestral and karmic diseases. Cause and effect is understood dispassionately when viewed from the perspective of this chakra. There is no emotional involvement. When activated and developed, it keeps the connection to your soul open and helps you access your karmic skills and abilities. It keeps the mind clear and focused, allowing soul input, ideas and intuition to flow freely. This chakra can assimilate scalar wave energy, bringing the subtle and physical bodies into alignment and activating DNA potential that is carried in the consciousness between the cell walls.

Physiology: Etheric and karmic blueprint, inherited and karmic diseases, DNA and RNA.

Sense: Purpose and true identity.

Positive qualities: Mindfulness. Living in the higher present moment.

Negative qualities: Living unconsciously propelled by your own past, ancestral or cultural imperatives.

Overactive/blown/spin too fast: If this chakra is blown you may be prey to wild imaginings and off-key intuitions.

Underactive/blocked/spin too slow: If this chakra is blocked your metaphysical abilities will be cut off from your conscious mind but may nevertheless affect your behaviour.

Typical dis-eases: are ancestral, karmic and beyond the physical although they may ultimately manifest as physical conditions.

Attachments: Past life and cultural or ancestral beliefs and soul imperatives.

The Three-chambered Heart Chakra
The sphere of deep compassion

The three-chambered heart chakra is an integrated chakra that resonates at a very high vibrational frequency. It is comprised of three parts: the 'traditional' heart chakra (see page 43), the higher heart (see page 70) and the heart seed (see below) and synthesises the qualities, potentials and dis-eases of those chakras. Opening and integrating the three-chambered heart is facilitated by having the soul star and stellar gateway chakras activated and connected to the earth star and Gaia gateway.

The Heart Seed
The sphere of soul remembrance

Location: Over the xiphoid process, at the tip of breastbone below the heart chakra.

The heart seed creates a connection to who you really are. It helps you to recall the reason for incarnation, encouraging you to be in spiritual service to humanity. Opening this chakra connects you to your soul purpose and how it fits into the overall divine plan. Placing a Brandenberg crystal here assists travel to the between-life state to ascertain your soul plan for the current lifetime and shows how to return to your original soul plan if you have deviated inappropriately. It also assists in renegotiating a past-its-sell-by-date soul purpose. It facilitates activating the karmic tools you have available to actualise your soul potential. When the heart seed is functioning optimally it brings with it a profound connection to your lightbody and multidimensional consciousness. The heart seed opens more easily when a connection has been made to the soul star, stellar gateway, and the alta major, Gaia gateway and earth star chakras are fully operational.

Physiology: The integrated physical and subtle energy systems.

Sense: Oneness.

Positive qualities: Compassionate, soul-orientated.

Negative qualities: Rootless, purposeless, spiritually lost.

Chakra connections: Forms part of the three-chambered heart chakra with the heart and higher heart.

Overactive/blown/spin too fast: When the heart seed chakra is blown heart energy and compassion cannot be integrated and expended appropriately. It can result in depletion and exhaustion from being overly compassionate, giving without consideration as to whether this is necessary or appropriate. It can result in spiritual interference with another person's journey and life lessons. It can also result in the spiritual martyr who feels hard done by, or in victimhood as others take advantage.

Underactive/blocked/spin too slow: If the heart seed is blocked, you are cut off from your purpose in incarnating and the kundalini cannot rise at a sufficiently high vibration to be incorporated into the lightbody as well as the physical, with consequent dis-ease occurring.

Typical dis-eases: Are those of depletion and disillusionment at a spiritual level.

Attachments: Parts of your soul left in other lives or dimensions. If you have left parts of yourself at past life deaths or traumatic or deeply emotional experiences, then these parts can be attached. They try to influence you to complete unfinished business that bears no relationship to the current life plan. They can be reintegrated and purified through the heart seed.

Note: The three-chambered heart chakra is opened and integrated as part of the Higher Chakra Integration that follows but the activation can be carried out as a stand-alone activity.

Higher Chakra Activation

This activation should be carried out with the basic chakras cleansed and open. Activate the chakras in order and do not rush the process. Open one at a time and give that chakra time to integrate into your entire chakra system before moving on to the next one. Allow yourself at least a week and probably longer to open and integrate all the higher chakras. And do this before activating kundalini. Remember to open all the chakras up to the new chakra before beginning a fresh activation. You can dowse to check whether a higher chakra has already opened and come on line, and when the opening and integration process is complete. This exercise is best done lying down as it facilitates placing the crystals and helps you to remain grounded.

Higher chakra activation stages

- Complete the chakra rebalancing and recharging exercise from page 75.
- Then open the higher chakras slowly and in order, first placing a large Smoky Elestial, Hematite or other grounding stone below your feet to anchor the energies, and a Selenite or Anandalite over

your head.

- Place a Gaia gateway chakra crystal on the Gaia gateway and feel it connect to the earth star to anchor all your energies bodies to the planet.
- Place a higher heart chakra crystal such as Rose Quartz, Danburite or Tugtupite over the higher heart chakra and leave it in place for two to five minutes. This chakra can be left open.
- Place a heart seed chakra crystal over the heart seed at the base of the breastbone and feel the influx of universal love that floods into the chakra and through your whole being. This chakra can be left open.
- When the higher heart and heart seed chakras have been opened, place crystals on all three heart chakras and feel the three-chambered heart chakra open and integrate. This chakra can be left open.
- Place a Preseli Bluestone or other cosmic anchor/soma chakra crystal such as Flint over the soma chakra. Open the chakra when you want to go journeying and close it when you want to stay in your physical body.
- Placing a high vibration crystal such as Selenite, Anandalite™ (Aurora Quartz), Rainbow Mayanite or Azeztulite on the soul star connects you to your soul and highest self. Invoke your higher self to guard it well. Be aware of its connection to the earth star. Close the chakra when not using the portal for journeying or guidance.

- Before opening the stellar gateway, invoke your guardian angel or other protective being to guard it well while you journey, meditate or seek guidance in other realms. Place Selenite, Anandalite, Phenacite, Rainbow Mayanite or other stellar gateway crystal to open the portal. Be aware of its connection to the Gaia gateway. Close the portal and the chakra when not in use.
- Use Anandalite™ (Aurora Quartz), Blue Moonstone or other alta major chakra crystal to activate the alta major chakra. Place in the hollow at the base of the skull. Feel the Merkaba within your skull connect up all the systems within. If you feel at all light-headed, take your attention down to the grounding stone at your feet. Remove the crystal and try again later.
- Dowse for the exact placement of the causal vortex, or use your hand to sense it. Place a causal vortex crystal above and behind your head. If you feel at all light-headed, take your attention down to the grounding stone at your feet. Remove the crystal and try again later.
- Remember to close each higher chakra when the activity is complete and open again before moving on to the next chakra activation.

The Subtle Energy Bodies

To understand how subtle bodies work, it helps if we imagine ourselves as a wave on the ocean. Our physical body is the very peak of that wave. Going deeper into the wave itself, we move away from the experience of time and space and the physical limitations of the body and into a broader definition of who we are, our emotions and our thoughts. If we go deeper still, a point is eventually reached where the edges of one wave cannot be differentiated from others: it stops being an individual wave and becomes part of the ocean.

– Simon and Sue Lilly, *Crystal Healing*

The physical body is surrounded and interpenetrated by subtle energy fields or 'bodies' that are usually called the aura or biomagnetic sheath. These bodies are linked through, but not limited to, specific chakras. The bodies are like blueprints that hold information, bio-memories and engrams from which the physical body will be constructed. The blueprints affect how the chakras function as well as physical, emotional and mental well-being. In some cases, blockages in the chakras will need to be released by healing the subtle energy body first. In other cases, clearing the chakra will result in a clearing of the subtle energy body. Medical science is slowly recognizing the existence of these bio-memory blueprints.

Bio-memories are memories that are locked into our cells. They carry hereditary memories, past life memories and memories that have become part of the very fiber of our current personality through constant repetition for years. Both physical and mental patterns can become part of our bio-memory. Bio-memories have the power to trigger physical actions like fight or flight. Mental states like depression and anxiety can quickly become part of our bio-memory if we are not careful. Bio-memories are not only unconscious, but are usually untraceable to any particular source incident.
– (original copyright holder unascertainable)

These bio-memories are also known as engrams, or engraved memories, and are:

biochemical changes that occur in neural tissues as the result of a powerful or persistent reaction to any situation. An engram is not an ordinary memory, but more like a photograph of the situation or event, complete with the emotional response that accompanied it. Engrams exist just below the level of our consciousness, influencing our emotional responses without our knowledge.

However, engrams are not just found in the physical

body. They also exist in the subtle bodies. You can picture these subtle energy bodies with their imprints as radiating out from the body in layers, with the chakras connecting them, each having a finer and more subtle vibration. But they are actually interlinked through multidimensional frequencies and interpenetrate each other. Crystals interact with the chakras and the blueprints to bring the bodies back into an appropriate harmony and equilibrium, and to heal energetic 'holes', energy loss, distortion or imprinted patterns that no longer serve you. Having these subtle bodies balanced and in harmony facilitates the flow of kundalini at higher vibrational levels.

Physical-etheric body

The physical subtle body, or etheric blueprint, tends to be close to the physical body and can often be seen with a psychic eye as a whitish aura around that body. It is a biomagnetic program and holds imprints of past life disease, injuries and beliefs which present life symptoms then reflect. It also holds subtle DNA that can be activated or switched off by behaviour and beliefs, and which in turn affects DNA in the physical body. It is connected through the seven traditional, lower frequency chakras on the body and the soma, past life, alta major and causal vortex.

Emotional body

The emotional body is created by emotions and feelings,

attitudes, heartbreaks, traumas and dramas, not only in the present life but in previous lives. Emotional dis-ease shows up as dark or distorted patches within the subtle emotional body and the solar plexus and heart chakras. The emotional body may contain engrams, bundles of energy that hold a deeply traumatic or joyful memory picture. Dis-ease in this body may also be reflected in the sacral and base chakras and the knees and feet which will act out insecurities and fears.

Mental body

The mental body is created by thoughts, memories, credos and ingrained beliefs from both the present and previous lives. It is connected particularly strongly through the throat and head chakras, but can be reflected in the lower body chakras also. This body holds the imprint of all that has been said or taught by authority figures in the past along with inculcated ideologies and points of view. It may need to be cleared and repro-grammed with perspectives more suitable to the current stage of spiritual growth so that it opens the way for evolution on all levels.

Karmic body

The karmic body or blueprint holds the imprint of all previous lives and the purpose for the present life. This means that it contains mental programs, physical imprints, engrams and emotional impressions and beliefs that you hold about yourself, many of which may be contradictory as they will arise from very different experiences in various lives. When the karmic body is healed, evolutionary intent can be actualised. This body is accessed through the past life, alta major and causal vortex chakras, but may also affect the soma, knee and earth star.

Ancestral body

The ancestral body holds all that you have inherited down your ancestral lines on both sides, everything your ancestors passed on to you at either the physical or more subtle levels. This can include family sagas, belief systems and attitudes, culture and expectations, traumas and dramas that shape your world. Healing sent back down the ancestral line to the core experience rebounds forward to heal the line going out into the future, making change possible. This body can be accessed through the soul star, past life, alta major, higher heart, earth star and Gaia gateway chakras, and can have a great deal to do with how much at home you feel on the planet and whether you are able to put your soul purpose into practice. You may need to release ancestral expectations before soul evolution can occur.

Planetary body

While you are in incarnation you also have a subtle energy body that links into the planet and the Earth's etheric body and meridians. This planetary body is also connected to the wider cosmos, the luminaries, planets and stellar bodies, and the outer reaches of the universe. Through this planetary body you are therefore connected into the wider whole. The planetary body is reflected in your birth chart and is accessed through the past life, alta major, causal vortex, soma, stellar and Gaia gateway chakras. Cosmic or soul dis-ease can be corrected through the planetary subtle body.

Spiritual or Lightbody

The spiritual or lightbody is an integrated, luminous, vibrating energy field consisting of the physical body and all the subtle energy bodies, plus the spirit or soul, connected through all the chakras but especially through the higher dimensional ones: soma, soul star, stellar gateway, Gaia gateway, alta major and causal vortex. It is an electromagnetic field of varying oscillation with integrated frequencies from the highest to the lowest: being light in all its varied manifestations. The body itself resonates with the universe, the universal mind and with your own soul or spirit. When the lightbody is activated, it can literally re-encode your DNA bringing out its highest potential and allowing your soul's purpose to manifest. When activated and integrated with kundalini it is the marriage of Shakti and Shiva discussed in the introduction.

To harmonize the subtle energy bodies
- Hold a piece of Anandalite or other subtle body harmonizer in your hand and sweep it at arm's

length from your feet up over your head and down to your feet at the back – if you find it difficult to reach ask a friend to assist. Then bring it up and over your head again and back to the floor.

- Sweep it from one side of your body to the other moving from your feet up over your head and down to your feet on the other side. Return to the first side.

- You may have to carry out several sweeps moving your arm closer in each time to integrate and harmonize all the subtle bodies with the higher dimensional energetic levels of the chakras.

To integrate and ground the chakra and subtle bodies connection

You will need a Shungite rod and a Selenite wand about a hand's breadth or a little longer but tumble stones may also work for you. Dowse or intuit which crystal to use on which knee. You may need to change sides halfway through the exercise as the energies integrate.

- Hold the Shungite rod in your left hand and place upright on your left knee. Dowse or intuit whether this is the correct side of the body. If not, change to the right hand and knee.

- Hold the Selenite rod in the other hand and place upright on the matching knee.

- Feel all the chakras and subtle energy bodies aligning.

- Feel yourself connecting your whole energy system to the Earth through your knee chakras.
- Hold in place for five–ten minutes until the energies integrate and harmonize.
- Change hands and knees if appropriate.

Balancing the Chakras and Subtle Energy Bodies with Crystals

Cleansing and rebalancing your chakras and maintaining your subtle bodies on a regular basis ensures your well-being and prepares you for kundalini awakening. Fortunately crystals will do this for you. You can either do a complete chakra cleanse and recharge, as below, or you can cleanse one chakra at a time if you particularly identify with the issue or qualities for that chakra or if there is a blockage. Placing crystals on the earth star chakra grounds or discharges the energies and reminds you to keep your physical body connected to the Earth. This cleanse-and-recharge will be particularly important as your energies shift to a higher vibration and new higher chakras come on line.

You can quickly check whether a chakra is open and functioning optimally by using a pendulum (see page 170). You can check the energetic state of your subtle bodies in the same way.

A simple but effective layout for bringing your body back into balance is to place a cleansed and activated crystal over each of your chakras – you can dowse or intuit which crystals are suitable, or follow the colours given below. Don't forget to check which of the minor chakras should be included (see diagram on page 21). Place an appropriate stone on each chakra and leave in place for 20–30 minutes.

Rebalancing and aligning layout

- Place Smoky Quartz, Flint, Hematite or other earth star crystal between and slightly below your feet. Picture light and energy radiating out from the crystal into the earth star chakra for two or three minutes and be aware that the chakra is being cleansed, its spin regulated, and its function re-energized.
- Place Red Jasper, Carnelian or other appropriate crystal on the base chakra. Picture light and energy radiating out from the crystal into the base chakra before moving through the physical body in a cleansing and revitalizing wave.
- Place Orange Carnelian, Golden or Orange Calcite or other appropriate crystal on your sacral chakra, just below the navel. Picture the radiating light and feel the cleansing and energizing process in the chakra and then through the subtle energy bodies.
- Place Yellow Jasper, Citrine or other appropriate crystal on your solar plexus. Picture the radiating light and feel the cleansing and energizing process in the chakra and then through

the emotional body.

- Place Green Aventurine, Rose Quartz or other appropriate crystal on your heart. Picture the radiating light and feel the cleansing and energizing process in the chakra and then through the subtle energy bodies.

- Place Blue Lace Agate, Lapis Lazuli or other appropriate crystal on your throat. Picture the radiating light and feel the cleansing and energizing process in the chakra and then through the mental body.

- Place Sodalite, Apophyllite or other appropriate crystal on your brow. Picture the radiating light and feel the cleansing and energizing process in the chakra and then in the subtle energy bodies.

- Place Amethyst, Quartz or other appropriate crystal on your crown. Picture the radiating light and feel the cleansing and energizing process in the chakra and then in your spiritual body.

- Now take your attention slowly from the soles of your feet up the midline of your body, feeling how each chakra has become balanced and harmonized and how each is connected to an energy body.

- Remain still and relaxed, breathing deep down into your belly and counting to seven before you exhale.

- Take your mind down to your base chakra and work up through each chakra again in turn. As you breathe in and hold, feel the energy of the re-energized chakra radiating out through your subtle bodies bringing each one into alignment with the others and with your physical body. You will build layer on layer of replenished and rebalanced subtle bodies so that your whole aura is in balance. If at any time you feel a blockage, simply breathe the light of the crystal into the site until it dissolves.

- When you feel ready, gather your crystals up, starting from the crown. As you reach the earth star chakra, be aware of the grounding cord anchoring you to the Earth and into your physical body.
- Cleanse your stones thoroughly (see page 173).

Cosmic and Shamanic Anchors

Cosmic and shamanic anchors hold you safely in incarnation during journeying, kundalini experiences and expanded consciousness. The anchoring begins with the grounding cord (see page 34) and then expands upwards into the cosmos. It links your connection to the Earth's core to the higher dimensions. The cosmic anchor is hooked way out in the cosmos at the tip of Sagittarius' arrow where the galactic centre is currently to be found. The cosmic anchor is a subtle energy tube-like conduit running down the central line of the body passing through the earth star deep into the Earth, attaching to the core. It links via the Gaia and stellar gateways and the soul star chakra upwards to the galactic centre. It solidifies your core energy and provides a grounding cable for the lightbody, enabling you to ride out Earth energy changes and assimilate downloads of high vibration energy and, where appropriate, grounding it into the Earth. The connection between the Gaia gateway and the stellar gateway directs kundalini flow back down into the subtle energy bodies rather than allowing it to shoot out from the top of the head and dissipate.

Setting the anchors in place

- Lie down and place a Hematite, Flint, Smoky Quartz, or Smoky Elestial Quartz or other grounding stone below your feet, and a Gaia Stone, Serpentine or other shamanic anchor stone a foot below that at the Gaia gateway (see Anchor page 216).
- Place a Preseli Bluestone, Selenite, Anandalite or one of the cosmic anchor stones about a foot above your head at the soul star and then another above that at the stellar gateway.
- Picture the earth star chakra about a foot beneath your feet opening like the petals of a water lily.
- Feel two roots growing from the soles of your feet down to meet at the earth star, passing through its crystal.
- The two roots twine together and pass down through the earth star into the Gaia gateway and its crystal. They then pass through the outer mantle and deep into the molten magma.
- When the entwined roots have passed through the magma, they reach the big iron crystal at the centre of the planet.
- The roots hook themselves around this ball.
- Allow the connection to pass up from the earth star through your feet, up your legs and the knee chakras and into your hips. At your hips the connection moves across to meet in the base chakra and from there to the sacral and the

dantien, and on up the spine to the top of your head to the soul star and stellar gateway chakras.

- Take your attention back to the earth star and be aware of its interdependent connection to the soul star chakra through the subtle energy bodies.
- Then take your attention to the Gaia gateway chakra and be aware that this has a second, inter-dependent connection to the stellar gateway chakra through the subtle energy bodies so that your whole body is encased within the anchors.
- From the stellar gateway a cosmic anchor rises high into the galaxy, passing the sun on its way to the galactic centre.
- When the cosmic anchor reaches the galactic centre it hooks around the top of the arrow in Sagittarius' bow.
- You are now held safely suspended between Earth and cosmos, anchored between the twin poles of Shakti and Shiva.

Harmonizing the Entire Energy System to a Higher Resonance

Once all your chakras are open, it is a simple matter to harmonize the whole subtle energy system and shift it to a higher level of functioning. Remember this needs to be carried out every time there's an energetic shift or whenever you begin to feel out of balance at an energetic level. It is especially essential before beginning kundalini activation. For the first harmonization layout, allow yourself at least an hour. It will take less time after that. Alternatively, you can use the 'figure of eight' layout (page 120) to harmonize the energy flows. Both harmonizations use earthy 'low' vibration stones in conjunction with high vibration ones. Earthy vibration stones tend to be more solid in colour and heavy in mass, such as the Jaspers and Tourmalines but this is not always so, and some such as Eye of the Storm (Judy's Jasper) combine both earthy and higher vibrations but may need different colours of the same stone. High vibration stones tend to be clearer such as variations of Quartz, Petalite, Phenacite, Anandalite and so on. But colour and type can play its part. Smoky Elestial Quartz, for instance, has a much higher vibration than Smoky Quartz and although Rose Quartz has a high vibration, Rose Elestial Quartz is much higher still, and some of the White Elestial or Nirvana Quartzes are even higher. (If you are in any doubt check with my *Crystal Encyclopedia*.)

Suggested harmonic resonance crystals

Earthy		High vibration	
Brown earthy:	Smoky Quartz	Brown high vibration:	Smoky Elestial
Red earthy:	Red Jasper	Red high vibration:	Triplite
Orange earthy:	Carnelian	Orange high vibration:	Orange Kyanite
Yellow earthy:	Yellow Jasper	Yellow high vibration:	Citrine
Green earthy:	Green Aventurine	Green high vibration:	Prasiolite
Pink earthy:	Pink Carnelian	Pink high vibration:	Pink Kunzite
Blue earthy:	Blue Lace Agate	Blue high vibration:	Indicolite Quartz
Purple earthy:	Amethyst	Purple high vibration:	Brandenberg
White earthy:	Milk Quartz	Clear high vibration:	Phenacite

Harmonizing the system

- Lie down comfortably.
- Begin by placing a crown chakra crystal such as Selenite above the crown, or Auralite 23 around your head. This opens the crown chakra so that if kundalini should spontaneously rise it will have somewhere to go.
- Place a grounding crystal such as Hematite, Smoky Quartz or Flint on the earth star and connect this to the Gaia gateway by placing a Smoky Elestial Quartz beneath it.
- Place 'low' vibration earthy stones on each of the traditional chakras at the back of your spine, and then place a harmonically resonant higher vibration crystal on each one on the front of your body (see suggestions above) so that the chakras are stimulated from both sides.
- Then open the higher vibration chakras by placing appropriate crystals. Be aware of the connection between the Earth and soul stars, the Gaia and stellar gateways.
- Feel the energy of the high vibration stones uplifting the resonance of your chakras and the subtle bodies so that they harmonize to a higher frequency.
- Lie for fifteen to twenty minutes feeling all the chakras and all the vibrational levels coming into balance and harmony.

Figure of eight

Drawing high vibration energy down into the body, the figure of eight layout synthesizes it with earth energy drawn up from the feet to create equilibrium, and ground the raised vibrations. It creates core energy solidity and integrates the subtle energy bodies, helping you to ride out and assimilate energetic changes.

You will need three cleansed and activated high vibration stones such as new generation Quartzes, Anandalite, Rainbow Mayanite or Green Ridge Quartz, and three cleansed and activated grounding stones (see page 261), and a synthesizing stone such as Elestial Quartz, Polychrome Jasper or Shiva Lingam.

The figure of eight layout

- Place a joining stone just below your navel.
- Place a high vibration crystal beside your body at shoulder level, one at the top of your head and one at shoulder level down the next side.
- Continuing the figure of eight shape, place a grounding stone level with your knees.

- Then one beneath your feet.
- Place the final one level with the one at your knees on the other side.
- Remember to complete the circuit back to the first stone placed using your mind or a wand.
- Leave the crystals in place for ten to fifteen minutes or until you feel completely balanced and grounded.
- Remove the crystals in the order you placed them.
- Stand up, stamp your feet and walk around.

The Earth's Chakras

Chakra points pour, radiate and give off energy by tapping into a variety of dimensional planes. They balance and regulate the electromagnetheric field of Earth to stabilize our planet's energy. They connect with Earth's vortices, working together as an energetic, crystalline grid around our planet.

– www.harmoniousearth.org

Just as there are chakras on the human body, so the Earth too has a chakra and subtle energy body system and energy circuit that spreads around its body linking ancient sacred sites and balancing its electromagnetic field. These chakras radiate over an area of many square miles. As with the physical body, the Earth's chakra system is being given an upgrade. Additional Earth chakras are becoming active to assimilate higher vibrational energies. These chakras boost and synthesize the major chakra system helping it to rebalance and uplift. Dobogókő in the Pilis Mountains of Hungary for instance has always been regarded as the heart chakra of that country. But now it, together with the Ganges in India, is boosting the somewhat depleted heart chakra energy of

Glastonbury in England. This in effect opens a three-chambered heart chakra to assimilate the new vibrations.

As with the human body, the Earth's chakras mediate energy. The points receive, radiate and give off energy by tapping into various dimensions and frequencies. Chakra points can easily become out of balance and require healing (see my *Earth Blessings: Using Crystals for Personal Energy Clearing, Earth Healing and Environmental Enhancement*). These chakra points can be used to bring balance, harmony and peace to the planet. Although there is no consensus as to exactly where these chakras are located, it is usually accepted that the main chakras are:

The Seven Major Earth Chakras

Base: Mount Shasta, California (alternatives: Grand Canyon; Sedona Black Mesa, USA)

Sacral: Lake Titicaca, South America (alternatives: Machu Picchu; Amazon River)

Solar plexus: Uluru, Australia

Heart: Glastonbury, England (alternatives: River Ganges, India; Dobogókő, Hungary)

Throat: Great Pyramid, Egypt

Third Eye: Kuh-e Malek Siah, Iran (alternative: Mount Fuji, Japan)

Crown: Mount Kailash, Tibet

In addition, American geomancer Robert Coon has identified other Earth chakras around the world, totalling 156, some of which are astrological:

Chakra	Location
1	Glastonbury (Tor) & Shaftesbury, England
2	Brandenburg Gate, Berlin, Germany
3	Montserrat – Placa de Catalunya, Barcelona, Spain
4	Island of the Sun, Lake Titicaca, Bolivia & Peru
5	Plaza Mayor, Lima, Peru
6	Rio Ucayli and Rio Maranon confluence, Iquitos, Peru
7	Uluru & Kata Tjuta, Australia
8	Nourlangie Rock, Kakadu, Northern Territory, Australia
9	Hamelin Pool, Gathaagudu (Shark Bay), Western Australia
10	Tirta Empul, Bali
11	Borobudur, Java, Indonesia
12	Mount Kinabalu, Sabah, Malaysia
13	Mount Kailas, Tibet
14	Karakul Lake – Ismail Samani, Pamirs, Tajikistan
15	Sundarbans, Sagar Island, Banyan Tree, Botanical Gardens, Kolkata, India/Bangladesh
16	Mount Shasta, California
17	Kachina Peaks Wilderness, Arizona, USA
18	Golden Hinde, Strathcona Provincial Park, Vancouver Island, Canada
19	El Tule – Palenque, Mexico
20	Laguna Corcovado, Corcovado National Park, Costa Rica

21 Cascada Cola de Caballo – Cerro de la Silla-Fuente de la Vida, Monterrey, Mexico
22 Mount Fuji, Japan
23 Mani San, Ganghwa Island, North & South Korea
24 Sefa Utaki, Nanjo City, Okinawa
25 Haleakala Crater, Hawaii
26 Pihemanu (Midway Atoll/Islands)
27 Mauna Loa & Mauna Kea, Hawaii
28 Lake Rotopounamu, New Zealand
29 Mount Panié, New Caledonia
30 Macquarie Island
31 Great Pyramid – Mount Sinai – Mount of Olives, Egypt – Israel – Palestine
32 Mecca, Saudi Arabia
33 Takht-e Soleiman (Throne of Solomon), Iran
34 Table Mountain, Cape Town, South Africa
35 The Pilansberg, South Africa
36 Mont-aux-Sources, Lesotho, South Africa
37 Sergiev Posad – Danilov, Moscow, Russia
38 Mount Konzhakovsky Kamen, Central Ural Mountains, near Serov, Russian
39 Mount Elbrus, Caucasus, Russia Republic of Georgia
40 The Buddha, Po Lin (Precious Lotus) Monastery, Lantau Island – Victoria Park, Hong Kong Island – Tai Mo Shan, New Territories; Hong Kong
41 Emei Shan – Gongga Shan – Leshan Buddha, Sichuan, China
42 Mt Pulag, Luzon Island, Philippines

43   Niagara Falls, USA/Canada

44   Pilot Knob State Park, Iowa, USA

45   Akimiski Island, James Bay, Canada

46   Mount Dimlang, Shebshi Mountains, Adamwa Plateau, Nigeria

47   Kaalom, Lake Chad, Chad

48   Isangila Falls, Democratic Republic of Congo (Zaire)

49   Marco Zero – Praca da Republica – Golden Chapel, Recife and Nova Jerusalem, Fazenda Nova, Brazil

50   Peter & Paul Rocks, Brazil, Atlantic Ocean

51   Parnaiba River Headwaters National Park – Capivara Mountain National Park – Confusion Mountains National Park, Piaui, Brazil

52   Plaza de Mayo, Buenos Aires, Argentina

53   Iguazu Falls, Argentina – Brazil – Paraguay, Concepcion, Paraguay and Parque Nacional Cerro Cora, Paraguay

54   Plaza de Armas – Cerro Santa Lucia – Cerro San Cristobal – Parque Forestal, Santiago, Chile

55   Jebel Toubkal, High Atlas Mountains, Morocco

56   Pico de Teide, Tenerife, Canary Islands

57   Chott el Djerid, Tunisia

58   Teatro Amazonas, Manaus and confluence of Rio Negro and Rio Solimoes, Brazil

59   Angel Falls, Venezuela

60   Lago Arari, Ilha de Marajo, Brazil

61   Christ the Redeemer, Corcovado Mountain, Rio de Janeiro, Brazil

62   Praca dos Tres Poderes, Brasilia, Brazil

63 Terreiro de Jesus, Pelourinho, Cidade Alta, Salvador, Brazil
64 High Tatra, Poland & Slovak Republic
65 Stortorget, Gamla Stan, Stockholm, Sweden
66 Mytikas – Plateau of the Muses, Mount Olympus, Greece
67 Arunachala Hill, southwest of Chennai, India
68 Piram Island, Gulf of Cambay – Narmada River, Gujarat, India
69 Adam's Peak, Sri Lanka
70 Uhuru Peak, Kibo, Kilimanjaro, Tanzania
71 Ukerewe Island, Tanzania – Mfangano Island, Kenya – Bugala Island, Uganda and Source of the Nile, Jinga, Uganda; Lake Victoria
72 Mt Nkungwe, Mahale Mountains National Park, Lake Tanganyika, Tanzania
73 Mount Belukha, Siberia & Tabun Bogdo, Altais, Mongolia
74 Uzynaral Strait, Ortasu, Sarymsek Peninsula, Lake Balkash, Kazakhstan
75 Cape Khoboy, Olkhon Island, Lake Baikal, Russia
76 The Hall of Supreme Harmony, Forbidden City, Beijing, China
77 Tai Shan, Shandong Province, China
78 Karakorum, Gobi Desert, Mongolia
79 Boulder, Colorado, USA
80 Mount Whitney, Death Valley
81 Cahokia Mounds, Illinois, USA
82 Three Sisters, Blue Mountains & Sydney, Australia

83   Mount Picton area, southwest Tasmania, Australia

84   Fraser Island, Queensland, Australia

85   Cerro de Puntas, Arecebo source, Puerto Rico

86   Great Exuma Island, Bahamas

87   Montego Bay, Jamaica

88   Mt Simpson – Mt Victoria, Owen Stanley Range, Papua New Guinea

89   Popomanaseu, Guadalcanal, Solomon Islands

90   Puncak Jaya – Danau Paniai, Pegunungan Maoke (Snow Mountains), Papua, Indonesia

91   Dakar, Senegal

92   Timbuktu, Lake Faguibine, Niger River, Mali

93   Fogo, Cape Verde Islands

94   Tsodilo Hill, Botswana

95   Kgalagadi Transfrontier Park, South Africa – Botswana

96   Great Zimbabwe Ruins, Zimbabwe

97   Khao Nan Mia, Surat Thani, Thailand

98   Lake Toba, Sumatra, Indonesia

99   Angkor Wat, Cambodia

100 Mount Tomaniivi, Vita Levu, Fiji

101 Tarawa Island, Gilbert Islands, Kiribati

102 Mount Silisili, Western Samoa

103 Denali (Mount McKinley), Alaska

104 Great Bear Lake, Canada

105 Fox Islands, Aleutian Islands

106 Mount Maromokotro, Massif de Tsoratanana, Madagascar

107 Piton des Neiges, Reunion Island

108 Morne Seychellois, Victoria, Seychelles

109 Mount Damavand, Iran

110 Vozrozhdeniya Island (Renaissance Island) in Aral Sea, Uzbekistan – Kazakhstan

111 Malek Siah Kuh, Zahedan, Iran

112 Klyuchevskaya Sopka, Kamchatka Peninsula, Russia

113 Sakhalin Island, from Terpeniya Bay to mountain north, near Poronaysk, Russia

114 Cherskiy, near juncture of Kolyma and Omolon Rivers, Siberia

115 Easter Island

116 Rano Aroi, Easter Island

117 Rano Koi, Easter Island

118 Reykjavik, Lake Thingvallavatn, Thingvellir, Iceland

119 Callanish, Isle of Lewis, Hebrides, Scotland

120 Nuuk, Greenland

121 Port Stanley, Falkland Islands

122 South Georgia (Island)

123 Lake Buenos Aires, Argentina

124 Wood Buffalo National Park, Alberta, Canada

125 Adelaide Peninsula

126 Bay of God's Mercy, Southampton Island, Canada

127 Ascension Island, Atlantic Ocean

128 St Helena Island, Atlantic Ocean

129 Mount Loma, Sierra Leone

130 Lena – Muna juncture, Siberia

131 Lake Ozero Taymyr, north of central Siberian

plateau

Earth's Kundalini

The Earth's kundalini flows in conjunction with the planet's energy circuit. For many years kundalini flowed along the Himalayas, centred around Mount Kailash, the world's crown chakra, flowing approximately east-west. In more recent times, however, the kundalini flow has moved and now flows north-south down the backbone of the Americas – the Rocky Mountains and the Andes. It is settling in but has created disturbances in the Earth's energy meridians that can be brought back into equilibrium through crystal earth healing (this is outside the scope of this book but see *Earth Blessing* in Resources).

What is Kundalini?

Kundalini energy is your dormant spiritual energy or your life force and it gives you life. It is a wondrous powerhouse of divine cosmic energy which resides in you and penetrates the whole universe... It is not only life energy, sexual energy but a healing energy for your mind, body and soul.
– (Too numerous to attribute)

Kundalini is a Sanskrit word meaning 'coiled like a snake'. But it may also be translated as 'serpent power' and kundalini energy is most often illustrated as one or two snakes rising up the spine to the crown chakra and above. According to yogic tradition, it resides in the base chakra coiled three and a half times around the sacrum, the 'sacred bone', awaiting activation. Awakening may take place through yoga, meditation, breathing, movement, chakra work or spontaneous eruption. It is a powerful and seemingly intelligent supra-spiritual life force that rises up the spine from the base chakra to the head. The term refers to a mechanism *and* an energy affecting both the physical and biomagnetic subtle bodies. It enlivens physically and spiritually, passing into and between each cell of the physical body and especially the brain, activating the hormonal system and higher consciousness. It is mediated by the chakras. Definitions and descriptions show that kundalini awakening is experienced uniquely by each individual but there are certain shared characteristics common to each kundalini event as a quick web search shows:[2]

Kundalini definitions

Goddess Shakti, also known as our Kundalini Energy, has finally come to Shiva, her eternal dance partner; their dance floor is the entire Universe. Enlightenment can be experienced in this place. Pure bliss, love and joy surround every part of you.

– Charles Brand, www.appealingenvironments.com

The power of kundalini is said to be enormous. Those having experienced it claim it to be indescribable. The phenomena associated with it varies from bizarre physical sensations and movements, pain, clairaudience, visions, brilliant lights, superlucidity, psychical powers, ecstasy, bliss, and transcendence of self. Kundalini has been described as liquid fire and liquid light.

– www.themystica.com

Symbolically, Shiva provides the stimulus to awaken the Shakti and draw her wisdom into union with him. When first awakened she is a furious serpent whose breath is fire. She proceeds upward from her nest within the root chakra via the path of 'Sarasvati' and soon the ego subsides.

Sarasvati is the goddess of eloquence and transcendent knowledge.
– Richard Rudis (Sonam Dorje)

Some people experience flashes of firelike heat, increased energy, or simply more pure aliveness. Their eyes might shine with an inner light, and they tend to activate others, much as a lit match lights other matches it comes close to. Eyes are not just light receptors. In advanced states of spiritual awakening, the eyes actually emit light.
– www.divineopenings.com

Kundalini, a Sanskrit word meaning 'circular power', is an individual's basic evolutionary force.
– Genevieve Lewis Paulson, *Kundalini and the Chakras*

The Luminous Cloud

According to Gopi Krishna, a noted kundalini expert, two forces come into play during kundalini activation. The nervous system begins to manufacture a more potent form of prana and this is delivered to the brain through the nervous system in the form of a 'luminous cloud'. This light-cloud stimulates an expansion of awareness and induces visionary experiences. At the same time a 'radiant nectar' rises up from the base chakra in a process that can be likened to a cosmic orgasm. The two streams of energy move into all the organs, systems and glands of the body to prepare it for an influx of higher consciousness. These two streams of energy may be responsible for many of the signs that kundalini is on the move.

Signals that Kundalini is stirring

A full Kundalini Awakening is a specific energetic experience that means all of the knots and issues of the psyche have been resolved. It's extraordinarily rare. Most people who experience some type of energetic experience are not experiencing a full awakening, but the beginnings of the movement of Kundalini in the body.

– www.theyogalunchbox.co.nz

Kundalini awakening is an ongoing process not a one-off event. It happens in stages, some big, some small. The signs differ not only with each method used to activate it but also each person. A classic Hindu kundalini experience induced by spiritual practice has been described by Gopi Krishna:

Suddenly, with a roar like that of a waterfall, I felt a stream of liquid light entering my brain through the spinal cord. Entirely unprepared for such a development, I was completely taken by surprise; but regaining my self-control, keeping my mind on the point of concentration. The illumination grew brighter and brighter, the roaring louder, I experienced a rocking sensation and then felt myself slipping out of my body, entirely enveloped in a halo of light. It is impossible to describe the experience accurately. I felt the point of consciousness that was myself

growing wider surrounded by waves of light. It grew wider and wider, spreading outward while the body, normally the immediate object of its perception, appeared to have receded into the distance until I became entirely unconscious of it. I was now all consciousness without any outline, without any idea of corporeal appendage, without any feeling or sensation coming from the senses, immersed in a sea of light simultaneously conscious and aware at every point, spread out, as it were, in all directions without any barrier or material obstruction. I was no longer myself, or to be more accurate, no longer as I knew myself to be, a small point of awareness confined to a body, but instead was a vast circle of consciousness in which the body was but a point, bathed in light and in a state of exultation and happiness impossible to describe.
– *Kundalini: Path to Higher Consciousness*

In a commentary on the experience, a noted yogic mystic suggests, however, that even this does not encompass a full kundalini experience. It is but a step along the way. And it is stated that there will be many such steps along the way. But it is the end goal of many Indian yoga practices and meditations.

Kundalini awakening occurs in a variety of spiritual experiences, however, not just those of the Eastern or indeed the religious persuasion. In religious experience it is perhaps the least recognized of the forces compelling the vision. When St Teresa of Avila said, "Let nothing perturb you, nothing frighten you. All things pass," she knew what she was talking about. Her years in the convent were punctuated by a severe illness that left her legs paralyzed for three years until a vision changed her life – but not her health which remained fragile. She had more than one kundalini experience, although she didn't call it that. To her it was an encounter with the divine. A mystical experience among many such, often accompanied by 'the grace of rapture' (a kind of spiritual orgasm), or 'auditory hallucinations', paranoid sensations of being pursued by the devil, swooning and seizures and twitches. She seems to have been through a whole gamut of symptoms. In her autobiography she recounts a typical experience:

I saw an angel very near me, towards my left side, in bodily form, which is not usual with me; for though angels are often represented to me, it is only in my mental vision. This angel appeared rather small than large, and very beautiful. His face was so shining that he seemed to be one of those highest angels called seraphs, who look as if all on fire with divine love. He had in his hands a long golden dart; at the end of the point methought there was a little fire. And I felt him thrust it several times through my heart in such a way that it passed through my very bowels. And when he drew it out, methought it pulled them out with it and left me wholly on fire with a great love of God.

She goes on to say how the pain in her soul spread into her body but it was accompanied by huge delight too.

She was transported, "consumed with the mingled pain and happiness." Typical kundalini side effects. Ultimately she was able to say:

> *In a state of grace, the soul is like a well of limpid water, from which flow only streams of clearest crystal. Its works are pleasing both to God and man, rising from the River of Life, beside which it is rooted like a tree.*

Individual experiences of the kundalini activation process vary considerably; some processes may be gentle and slow, others dramatic and rapid, but signs and experiences that have been reported include in no particular order:

Signs and symptoms

- the sense that something transformative is happening internally
- deep dissatisfaction or a yearning for inner development
- feeling different, yearning for something *other*, not fitting in
- altered states of consciousness
- energy flowing or vibrating within the body
- spontaneous bodily movements or breathing patterns
- energetic sensations like electricity in the body or internal lightning bolts
- shaking and jerking in the body, totally out of

conscious control
- sensation of insects or snakes crawling on the body, often along the spine
- head feels full of intense pressure, 'fit to burst'
- waves of intense pleasure or bliss, sometimes leading to orgasm
- extreme emotional fluctuations or mood swings
- inner sensations of light, sound, severe cold or intense heat in the spine and chakras
- heightened inner or outer awareness
- moments of bliss
- flashes of insight
- increased sensitivity
- 'celestial music' or music of the spheres is heard with the inner ear
- special abilities, capacities, and talents emerge
- exceptional human experiences (EHEs) occur: visions, out-of-body experiences and so on
- psychic phenomena
- sensory overload – sounds, light, noise, touch become too much
- internal sounds audible only to the experiencer
- psychological issues rise to the surface as catharsis
- atypical sensations or sensitivities appear and disappear
- an interest in spiritual growth or in metaphysics or the esoteric
- compassion and a desire to help others
- spiritual realization

- heightened periods of creativity

Note: Some people experience migraine headaches from alta major chakra and/or kundalini activation. This is generally caused by too much energy congregating in the head. Placing a releasing crystal on the crown, third eye, soma chakra and/or base of your skull quickly discharges this. Open the chakra, picturing a flower that unfolds, releasing the excess energy into the crystal. Keeping a grounding crystal at your feet during activation processes also assists as does placing crystals at the Gaia and stellar gateways before commencing any activity that may awaken kundalini.

The Anatomy of Kundalini

*The Kundalini process may seem to be something totally
outside of our current understanding of how the body
works. But in fact, it is the activity of this mechanism, in a
reduced or limited form, which maintains and controls the
overall functioning of our body at all times.*
– www.icrcanada.org

In traditional, conventional, Western understanding, the
brain and nervous system, including the spinal cord, are
composed of sensory and motor neurons. These neurons
are activated by electrochemical processes transmitted
from cell to cell via synapses. Thoughts are generated in
the brain and pass, as electrical impulses, along the
neural pathways to affect the body. Mind or
consciousness has, for the most part, been seen as a
product of the brain. These concepts are, however, now
being challenged. It is being recognized that thoughts
and memory can be stored in the cells and muscles of the
physical body and its energy systems, rather than the
brain, and that consciousness can operate even after
brain death and so cannot be a product of the brain. The
brain is a carrier for consciousness and a mechanism

through which it can affect the physical level of being. (For a more thorough discussion on the nature of consciousness and current research see my *Book of Psychic Development*.) In the esoteric traditions of India, however, *prana* is recognized as the mechanism through which brain activity occurs. We are, therefore, looking at subtle anatomy that interacts with and stimulates the physical body but which has its own energetic and evolutionary vehicle.

> *Contemporary spiritual literature often notes that the chakras, as described in the esoteric kundalini documents, bear a strong similarity in location and number to the major endocrine glands, as well as nerve bundles called ganglions. One speculation is that the traditional practices have formalized a method for stimulating the endocrine glands to work in a different mode which has a more direct effect on consciousness, perhaps ultimately by stimulating the release of DMT by the pineal gland, which may be analogous to the 'pineal [third eye] chakra'.*
> – Tenzin Gyurme, *S-Alchemy*[3]

Subtle terminology

Although the Indian yogis have long had a language with which to describe the kundalini experience and its physiological mechanism and effects, it is difficult to translate this into terminology we in the West can easily understand. How are we to understand statements such as "three knots or *granthis* are broken" without a thorough grounding in the Vedic view of subtle anatomy. This is a very different view of how the body functions. Even within the Indian descriptions the terminology may have different interpretations. Prana may be called bioenergy or bio-plasma in the West but is it the same as kundalini? Prana is most often perceived as being a psycho-spiritual life force concentrated and stored in the sexual organs and the base and sacral chakras. Under normal circumstances a limited amount rises up the spine to the brain. However, during kundalini awakening, a much greater and more potent concentration floods the system. Ideally, it has first been enhanced or transmuted to a higher vibrational energy *and the physical body has been prepared to receive it.* If this transformation does not take place, very unpleasant side effects can result (see page 155).

The mechanism for kundalini flow is the *nadis*. But the *nadis*, subtle channels, are difficult to characterise. They are described as:

astral tubes made up of astral matter that carry psychic currents. The Sanskrit term 'Nadi' comes from the root 'Nad' which means 'motion'. It is through these Nadis (Sukshma, subtle passages) that the vital force or Pranic current moves or flows. Since they are made up of subtle matter they cannot be seen by the naked physical eyes and you cannot make any test-tube experiments in the physical plane. These Yoga Nadis are not the ordinary nerves, arteries and veins that are known to the Vaidya Shastra

(Anatomy and Physiology). Yoga Nadis are quite different from these.
– Sivananda Saraswati, www.sivananda.org

So, in the conventional Western medical view, as they can't be measured or seen, *nadis* are unlikely to exist. Fortunately Western medical science is beginning to move away from such a literal interpretation of the body as more of the underlying processes of the transference of impulses and sensations through the nervous system become apparent.

There is some correlation between Western and Eastern anatomy, and that of the physical and subtle energy bodies. The *nadis* and their association with the physical body have been described by a yogi as:

On either side of the spinal cord run the sympathetic and para-sympathetic cords, a double chain of ganglia [a collection of nerve cells]. These constitute the autonomic system which supplies nerves to the involuntary organs, such as heart, lungs, intestines, kidneys, liver, etc., and controls them... [the] sympathetic system stimulates or accelerates, [the] para-sympathetic system retards or inhibits... The left and the right sympathetic chains are connected by filaments. These cross from the right to the left side and vice versa... [However the] Ida and Pingala Nadis are not the gross sympathetic chains. These are the subtle Nadis that carry the Sukshma Prana. In the physical body these tentatively correspond to the right and left sympa-

thetic chains. Ida starts from the right testicle and Pingala
from the left testicle. They meet with Sushumna Nadi at
the Muladhara Chakra and make a knot there.
– www.yoga-age.com

From there on, the description of the process becomes
more complex. But we can see that the *nadis* in the subtle
bodies correspond approximately to the nervous system
in the physical body. The *granthis* correspond to specific
ganglions, nerve centres that are placed along the spine
at the position of the chakras and at the third eye. The
central channel that carries cerebrospinal fluid up and
down the spine has a similar correlation to the *sushamna*
channel. However, these are operating at an energetic
level that impacts on the physical. They are not part of
the physical body itself.

What is clear is that kundalini has a profound effect
on the hormonal and chemical secretions of the brain
and body *and* on metaphysical perception and
consciousness. So, although it may not be possible to
completely reconcile the two systems, we can utilise
what we know of the chakras and subtle energy bodies,
and harness this to the energetic resonance and healing
effect of crystals.

The Crystal Palace

Taoists call the center of the brain between the pineal and
the pituitary 'the Crystal Palace'… It's said that when the
pineal gland is activated it becomes illuminated like a

*thousand suns... When the Crystal Chamber is lit
transcendental vision occurs.*
– www.alchemylab.com

The pineal and pituitary glands are two of the major hormone producing sites in the brain, under the control of the puppet master the hypothalamus at the centre. The pineal gland is located where the 'oldest' region of the brain, the cerebellum, meets the 'newer' cerebral cortex at the top of the spinal cord. (This is one of the anchor and activation points for the alta major chakra, see page 89.) The pituitary sits slightly forward in the brain on the other side of the spinal cord.

The pineal gland mediates the circadian rhythm, the sleep-waking cycle, through the production of melatonin but it also produces dimethyltryptamine. DMT. 'The spirit molecule' is coming to be recognized for its role in exceptional human experiences such as precognition, intuition, out-of-body experiences and the like. The physical shape of the pineal bears an extraordinary resemblance to Egyptian pictures of the Eye of Horus. It is the 'all seeing eye', the third eye chakra that is the linkage point between the spiritual and physical worlds. As more is being scientifically uncovered as to the role of the pineal, it has been found that this gland is in itself crystalline, containing hydroxyapatite (the 'brain sand' previously mentioned). The energies of healing crystals can entrain with this natural brain-crystal, bringing it into balance and activating its metaphysical abilities as well as elevating the frequency of the brain. This metaphysical gland acts as a multidimensional energy structure into which higher vibrational energies can anchor.

Although only the size of a pea, the pituitary gland is known as the 'master gland' as it plays a vital role in regulating many functions of the physical body and ensuring well-being. It also controls other glands such as the thyroid and adrenals, all of which may be affected by uncontrolled kundalini rise and the resulting hormonal flood.

The pineal and pituitary glands are housed in an area of the brain known esoterically as the 'the crystal palace'. That major nerves and blood vessels which serve the eyes and middle ear run alongside this area may account for some of the metaphysical symptoms of kundalini awakening. As may raised levels of psychedelic and mood enhancing hormones, such as dopamine and phenylethylamine, which are released during the experience. But the overall goal, certainly as far as the yogis are concerned, is the raising of consciousness to an expanded level. This is one of the major benefits of kundalini awakening.

Benefits of Awakened Kundalini

One of the first results of research on Kundalini, in my view, would be to show that the human brain is already evolving towards a higher predetermined state of consciousness, a state that has been the crowning vision of the mystics and the prophets.

– Gopi Krishna

As little actual scientific study has been done on the effects of kundalini much of the information comes from anecdotal evidence and hundreds of years of esoteric reportage especially in Vedic literature. Numerous reports reveal that benefits include:

Kundalini benefits

- being more fully present in daily life
- unconditional self-love
- handling life with grace and ease
- increased physical, emotional, mental and spiritual well-being
- more aware of sensations, bodily functions and energy levels
- bio-memory and biometric changes

- spontaneous healing of chronic conditions
- increased cellular energy
- huge sense of release from previous burdens and baggage
- increased emotional intelligence and mental agility
- sharper focusing and problem-solving abilities
- extremely rapid multiprocessing
- higher alertness levels
- better short-term memory
- experiences of cosmic consciousness
- greater spiritual awareness
- enlightenment
- amplified intuition
- inner peace
- transcendental states of awareness
- superlucidity
- heightened sensitivity at all levels
- increased paranormal/metaphysical abilities
- increased empathy and compassion
- activation of the spiritual rather than the personal will
- change in vibrational frequency
- slower aging
- ability to catalyse others

The Nithyananda Dhyanapeetam Study

A study carried out in 2011 with over 600 participants on a 21-day yoga intensive awakening workshop assessed the effects of kundalini activation and personal initiation sessions. The study was apparently based on a similar study conducted by Jeffery A. Dusck at Harvard Medical School (allegedly published in July 2008 but so far untraceable). Recordings were taken on the first and eighteenth day of the yoga intensive. Unfortunately, however, in the online report there is no record of the scientists and/or medical researchers who actually conducted the study (to follow up, see www.nithyananda.org); and it has not been peer reviewed so, although much quoted, it awaits verification. Nevertheless, the report makes interesting reading as it confirms the reported anecdotal evidence; but I leave you to read it and draw your own conclusions. The parameters studied included:

- Cellular energy levels
- Physical health and immunity levels
- Psychological and emotional health
- Neurological changes in the brain
- Genetic transformation, if any
- Expression of any extraordinary abilities

Findings

It is reported that, from blood samples taken, 100 per cent of participants aged over 50 experienced a drastic increase in cellular energy. In the overall group, rapid recovery from a range of physical ailments was observed, also indicating enhanced immunity levels, and participants also recorded lowering of fasting blood sugar, lower BMI and improvement in psychosomatic illnesses and autoimmune diseases, decreased dependency on medication and an enhanced sense of well-being, clinical improvement in rheumatoid arthritis, fibromyalgia and other chronic pain conditions, recovery from asthma and significant improvements in memory. It would therefore appear that the initiations and kundalini activation had resulted in very significant improvements.

You will find links to one or two other ongoing studies in the Resources section at the end of this book.

The Downside of Uncontrolled Kundalini Rise

There is much dumping of adrenaline into the body and frying your system is a real possibility and danger.
– Dr Glenn Morris

Kundalini awakening is probably the most common type of spiritual emergency. The Spiritual Emergence Network Newsletter reported that 24% of their hotline calls concerned kundalini awakening experiences.
– www.spiritualcompetency.com

Kundalini awakening can be extremely uncomfortable, especially if you're not aware of what is happening. Many 'new age children', such as the indigo and crystal kids, are born with high levels of unmediated kundalini energy. This may explain why many of them find it so difficult to adapt to living within a dense physical body. It can be mistaken for all manner of physiological and psychological disturbances. Spiritual activities such as meditation and shamanic journeying may trigger it prematurely. This is particularly so if the subtle energy bodies and chakra connections are unprepared, weak, 'toxified', or unbalanced. Intense energy work, trauma or abuse, childbirth, drug use, excessive sexual experiences, emotional shocks, mental overload, stress, yoga practice or life events and so on can also activate kundalini power to involuntarily flood the energy systems before they are prepared to assimilate it.

The level at which the energy systems are blocked – physical, emotional, ancestral, psychological and so on – will determine the side effects. The resultant kundalini clearing may be experienced as a reactive depression, for instance, when the psychological level or 'mental chakras' are blocked. When the physical level or belly chakras are blocked, the body expresses the clearing as a physiological symptom. This clearing occurs through the nearest available chakra or organ. As Genevieve Lewis Paulson explains:

> *Kundalini will look for the most open area or chakra to 'escape' through if the body is not ready to receive its energies, blowing open a particular area or chakra and tending to pull all energies towards that spot, as if to a black hole.*

She highlights how important it is to release memories, emotions, feelings and blockages during the kundalini cleansing process and not suppress them further. When they arise, stay with it and let them move through you. The secret is to acknowledge and feel without becoming enmeshed and trapped in the feelings. Fortunately crystals move the energy of a feeling or blockage from where it is stuck and encourage it to flow once again until it is assimilated or eliminated. Placing a crystal on the back of a chakra or out in the subtle energy body at the rear moves the focus from the front of the body, where the dis-ease is usually felt most strongly, and allows the toxic or blocked energy to expand and release. This is where crystals are such a useful tool as they gently facilitate release, transmutation and rebalancing.

Adverse reactions and possible side effects

Traditionally, kundalini awakening was carried out in carefully monitored stages under the guidance of an expert teacher. Those who undergo an involuntary kundalini experience before the chakras and the physical and energy bodies have been fully prepared may suffer from symptoms which vary from the comparatively minor to verging on psychotic. Therefore it is wise to undertake kundalini activation in slow, careful stages ensuring that you have fulfilled each preparatory step by activating and balancing each of the chakras first, and integrating the subtle energy bodies. The experience can then be grounded into everyday reality and into cells of the physical body that are ready to receive and assimilate the influx of energy. Even when kundalini rise is voluntary and controlled, the cleansing process that precedes assimilation and healing may be extremely uncomfortable and may create a catharsis. Fortunately there are crystals that will release, regulate and return to equilibrium any adverse reactions – see the A–Z Directory.

Physiological

- insomnia, abnormal sleep patterns
- adrenal overload
- breakdown of the immune system
- breakdown of the nervous system
- bladder infections or diarrhoea
- digestive upsets
- muscular inflexibility
- menopause-like symptoms
- back, shoulder or neck pain
- arrhythmia (irregular or abnormal heart rhythm)
- palpitations
- dizziness
- fainting
- shortness of breath
- chest discomfort
- debilitation and lethargy
- severe headache or migraine
- tremors, twitches and chills
- fierce cold or hot flashes
- overstimulation/sensitivity of the senses
- Meniere's Disease
- tinnitus
- ME
- diabetes

- restless leg syndrome
- severe weather sensitivity

Psychological

- disorientation
- difficulty in dealing with everyday life
- ego inflation
- depression
- excessive mood swings/bipolar
- visual effects – visions, colours, past life glimpses
- sexual obsession or impotence
- mental confusion or overload
- memory loss or distortion
- disintegration of the psyche
- erratic behaviour
- loss of control
- retreat into fantasy and phobias
- serious psychosis

Metaphysical

- psychic overwhelm
- uncontrollable visions
- overwhelming past life memories
- uncontrolled out-of-body experiences
- losing your way on the astral plane

Spiritual

- loss of spiritual connection
- soul loss

You will find crystals to help you rebalance and heal these symptoms listed in the A–Z Directory.

Activating Kundalini with Crystal Assistance

Named after the Sanskrit for fire, Agnitite is a hematite-based Quartz that has been designated one of the highest vibration stones for spiritual transformation and transfer of higher dimensional energies. This powerful Quartz lights your inner fire. When placed on the base chakra, power flashes up the spine and shoots out of the top of your head to open the higher crown chakras before falling back through the body to fertilize your cells. It needs to be used with care unless you have already worked with high vibration crystals. Too rapid a kundalini rise causes physical and spiritual imbalances, 'blowing your mind' or your cells causing physical disturbances, so other stones such as Mohawkite or Smoky Elestial Quartz may be needed to assist with integration and grounding of these new energies. Having heightened the frequency of the physical body, Agnitite integrates the lightbody and raises the energetic resonance of the whole.

– Judy Hall, *Crystal Bible volume 3*

Once all the chakras have been cleansed, activated and

balanced, and the subtle bodies aligned, there are various techniques that can assist with raising kundalini. The simplest of these is a combined breathing and crystal placement exercise that transmutes prana into a higher frequency energy. It expands the microcosmic orbit (see page 78), taking the energy out to the subtle bodies as well as through the front and back of the physical spine and the chakras. It can be worked in gentle stages so that each chakra has assimilated the rise and adapted its frequency before moving on to the next. The energy rise will be subtle at first but over time can become orgasmic, a rush of bliss moving up your spine. This is when you need to keep control of the energy, directing its course with the crystal and with your mind.

It may be sensible to use an earthier stone such as Poppy Jasper or Serpentine when first undertaking the exercise and then move on to higher vibrational stones such as Kundalini Quartz or Anandalite as the channels open. Remember to put your shamanic and cosmic anchors in place, and position an appropriate crystal above your head at the stellar gateway and one at your feet at the Gaia gateway so that the energy is able to flow back down and circulate rather than blasting out of the top of your head. Focusing your attention on each chakra in turn helps the energy to rise. Lying down makes placing a crystal above your head and below your feet easier if you are working alone. You could sit or stand and ask a helper to assist by holding a stellar gateway crystal above your head.

As it can be difficult to reach around behind you to the chakras on the back of your spine, it can be useful to have someone assist this process by moving the crystal for you. However, you will need to guide them as to the speed with which they move the crystal. This can be done by asking them initially to move it in time with your breathing – and you can use your hand to indicate this. Moving it up as you inhale and holding it still as you exhale. An intuitive assistant will soon attune to your breathing pattern and move the crystal accordingly.

If you do not have an assistant and cannot reach your back when lying on your side, you can move the crystal up the front of your body but use the power of your mind to visualize and *feel* the energy moving up the back of your spine.

Raising the kundalini

You will need:

A grounding stone such as Flint, Smoky Quartz or Smoky Elestial Quartz.
A stellar gateway crystal such as Azeztulite, Phenacite, Selenite or Serpentine.
A kundalini activating crystal such as Anandalite, Kundalini Quartz, Poppy Jasper, Red Amethyst, Red Jasper, Sedona Stone or Serpentine.

• Place a grounding stone at the Gaia gateway chakra or between your feet if sitting or standing.

- Place a stellar gateway crystal above your head.
- Put your shamanic and cosmic anchors in place (see page 115).
- Hold your kundalini activating crystal over your base chakra.
- Clench your perineum and anus.
- Breathe deeply down into the base chakra at the base of your belly until you can feel the kundalini energy stirring and meeting the energy of the crystal.
- When the energy begins to move, as you breathe in pull it up the back of your spine towards the sacral chakra. As you breathe out clench and hold the energy in place, slowly moving the crystal upwards as you do so. Allow the crystal to accompany the energy, do not force it.
- Continue to inhale and pull the energy up; exhale and clench, holding the energy in place, and then raising it up once more until it reaches the sacral chakra.
- Inhale deeply into your sacral chakra and let it fill with kundalini and the energy from the crystal. Clench and hold it there as you breathe out. Repeat four or five times.
- Then move your crystal up towards your dantien as you inhale deeply and pull the energy up to your dantien. As you exhale, clench and hold the energy so that it fills the dantien.
- Breathing deeply and slowly moving your crystal, let the energy flow up to the solar plexus. As you

exhale, clench and hold the energy so that it fills the sacral chakra.

- From here it is a small step to the heart seed chakra. Breathe into your spine level with the base of your breastbone and allow the kundalini energy and that of the crystal to flow into the heart seed.

- As it does so, feel how the heart chakra opens to receive the kundalini. Let your heart fill with the energy. Breathe deeply into your heart and feel how it opens to allow the kundalini to flow up into the higher heart chakra so that the three-chambered heart chakra is on fire with kundalini. Stay with this energy, breathing gently and letting it find its point of equilibrium. Do not hurry the process.

- When the energy has stabilized, continue inhaling and exhaling in a regular rhythm, bringing the energy and the crystal up to the rear of the throat chakra. Breathe deeply into the throat chakra and feel the kundalini meet the energy of the crystal and fill and open your throat.

- Move the crystal and the kundalini energy up and over the back of your head until you reach a point level with the third eye. Continue breathing into that point until the energy stabilizes.

- Then breathe into your crown chakra and pull the energy into it. Holding your crystal on the crown, continue breathing until the crown chakra fills with kundalini.

- Inhaling and exhaling in a gentle rhythm, take the

crystal down the front of your body, pausing at each chakra and feeling the energy connect until you reach the base chakra once more.

- Be aware that you have a circuit of kundalini energy running up the back of your spine and down the front of your body.

- After you have completed a few circuits, when you reach the crown chakra allow the kundalini to move up through the soul star connecting with that chakra. Feel it flow from there down to the earth star beneath your feet and then up your shamanic anchor roots into your feet, legs and hips. Move it across to the base chakra and begin the circuit again.

- After several more circuits, allow the kundalini to reach the stellar gateway chakra and cascade down through your energy bodies until it reaches the Gaia gateway chakra. Bring it up to the earth star and up around your energy bodies.

- Feel how the flow through your body extends out and meets the flow through your subtle energy bodies. This connection is particularly strong at each chakra. Move your crystal in turn to each of the chakras.

- You will then have a two-way flow, up and down the spine and up and down the energy bodies, which is connected through the chakra vortexes.

- Once the flow has been activated and is in harmony, simply rest in the flow, allowing the energy to permeate every pore of your being at every level.

- Store the energy in your base chakra or dantien when the exercise is complete. Spiral the energy into the chakra using your crystal and visualize folding the 'petals' of the chakra over to close it. See close down page 165.

If at any time you feel discomfort or distress, hold the crystal still and breathe into the chakra until a release is felt. It may then be sensible to leave the session at that point until the energy has stabilized and return to it later. In which case, store the kundalini in the base chakra or dantien by visualizing the energy spiralling in and the chakra closing over it (see To close down page 165). If you have someone assisting you, it can be helpful if they hold a Smoky Quartz, Obsidian or Flint crystal over the chakra to absorb anything that needs to be released (don't forget to cleanse the crystal afterwards).

The exercise can also be carried out with you lying on your side and a helper massaging the back or front of each of your chakras with a crystal. Your assistant then moves on to the next chakra when you indicate that the energy, which you have been pulling up with your breath as before, has reached the next chakra. When all the chakras have been filled and the kundalini is flowing through the subtle energy bodies, huge sweeps of Anandalite or Serpentine from the feet up to the head and back help the energy to stabilize.

To close down

- Allow your breathing to quieten and rest the crystal over your dantien or base chakra.
- Feel the kundalini spiralling down into the chakra and the chakra closing over it like petals folding in. If necessary, hold a piece of Flint over the chakra to lock it closed for the time being.
- Take your attention down to your feet and ensure that your grounding root is in place.
- Focus your attention into the earth star chakra, and feel it holding you gently in incarnation and connected to the Earth.
- If you have been sitting or lying, stand up and feel your feet in contact with the Earth.
- Close the higher chakras above your head by visualizing them folding in on themselves like a flower closing, or place a closing crystal such as Flint over them.
- Check whether any of your chakras need to be slowed down or regulated and, if so, place an appropriate crystal over them for a few moments.
- Move around, have a hot drink and, preferably, walk on the earth with bare feet to ensure you are fully grounded and any excess energy discharged.

The same process can be used for a chakra close down, omitting spiralling the kundalini into the dantien or base chakra.

Crystal Essentials: Choosing and Taking Care of Your Crystals

It's tempting to rush straight into the healing work, but let's look at the basics first as it makes your crystal experience much more productive. For instance, crystals carry the energy of everyone who touches them and many draw off toxic vibes but all require regular cleansing. Crystals want to cooperate with you so setting an intention is vital. And, finally, there is one small secret that makes your crystal work so much more potent.

– Judy Hall, *Earth Blessings*

166

A few simple steps when you begin makes using crystals for chakra balancing or kundalini awakening a much more effective tool.

Finding your prescription

Every body is different. Quite literally. Each person has their own unique vibration and bioenergetic field. Everyone is at a different stage of their energetic and spiritual evolution. So there is no 'one stone fits all' remedy. Therefore you need to find the crystal or combination of crystals that works best for you. The best way to select your crystals and to identify where to place them is to dowse for them or choose them intuitively (see page 169). Most entries in this directory offer a choice of crystals to assist a particular chakra or issue. While all the stones listed in the directory could potentially help you, selecting the right crystal is crucial if you are to obtain maximum benefit and the fastest relief or most effective harmonizing. Some crystals have a much finer vibration than others, working from the etheric to adjust the physical; and some work at a physical level so you may need to use a series of crystals or combine them.

You may find that you are instinctively drawn to a particular stone and it may be one that you already have in your collection. If so, try this one first.

You can also dowse when purchasing a healing crystal, either by allowing your fingers instinctively to pick the right stone from a selection – the right one will 'stick' to them – or using a pendulum or finger dowsing (see page 169). All methods use the ability of your intuitive body-mind connection to tune into subtle vibrations and to influence your hands. A focused mind, trust in the process, carefully worded questions and a clear intent supports your dowsing and your healing.

Framing your question

An answer brings no illumination unless the question has matured to a point where it gives rise to this answer which thus becomes its fruit. Therefore learn how to put a question.

– Egyptian Proverb

Framing your question with precision is essential if you are to achieve the most beneficial result. Your questions need to be unambiguous and capable of a straight 'yes' or 'no' answer. They also need to be asked with serious intent. An irresponsible approach or a frivolous question is unlikely to reveal anything of lasting benefit, and could actually do harm as crystals are powerful tools that pick up and amplify your thoughts. They should be treated with respect.

Take time to prepare yourself to ask the question. Sit quietly for a few moments, bringing your focus away from the outside world and quietening your mind. Word your question carefully. If, for instance, you ask: "Is this the right crystal for me?" the answer could well be 'yes' but it may not refer to the chakra or condition you are dealing with at that precise moment. It could indicate a crystal that would give you long-term benefit for an, as yet, unrecognized issue or potential energy shift that exists at an emotional, mental or soul level. That crystal could well be of value to you in the long term, but it would not heal the immediate situation, or work on the specific chakra. You need to be specific. If you are finger dowsing (see page 169), ask: "Is [name of crystal] the best and most appropriate crystal to balance my sacral chakra at this time?" If you are pendulum dowsing (see page

170), ask: "Please show me the best and most appropriate crystal to balance my sacral chakra now."

Dowsing

There are several methods of dowsing so try them in turn until you find the one that works best for you and then practise to refine your technique. Dowsing for solutions works best in an energetically clear space.

Finger Dowsing

Finger dowsing answers 'yes' and 'no' questions quickly and unambiguously, and can be done unobtrusively in situations where a pendulum might provoke unwanted attention. This method of dowsing works particularly well for people who are kinaesthetic, that is to say their body responds intuitively to subtle feelings, but anyone can learn to finger dowse. It is useful for checking whether a chakra is open, closed or blocked but it is not so easy to ascertain whether the chakra is spinning in the appropriate direction at a suitable speed.

To finger dowse

To finger dowse, hold the thumb and first finger of your right hand together (see illustration). Loop the thumb and finger of your left hand through to make a 'chain'. Ask your question clearly and unambiguously – you can speak it aloud or keep it within your mind. Now pull gently but firmly. If the chain breaks, the answer is usually 'no'. If it holds, the answer is usually 'yes' – but check by asking your name in case your response is reversed.

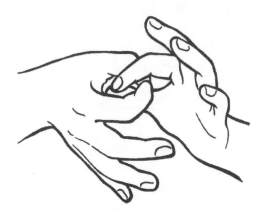

Body dowsing

As bodies are extremely sensitive to changing vibrations you can use your hands to dowse the chakras. Open your palm chakras (see page 60), extend them forwards with your palms turned up and facing out. Pass your hand up the spine or front of the body and allow yourself to sense whether a chakra is closed or open, whether it is buzzing or whizzing out of control, or whether it is in balance.

Pendulum dowsing

If you are familiar with pendulum dowsing, use the pendulum in your usual way. If you are not, this skill is easily learned.

To pendulum dowse

To pendulum dowse, hold your pendulum between the thumb and forefinger of your most receptive hand with about a hand's length of chain hanging down to the pendulum – you will soon learn what is the right length for you. Wrap the remaining chain around your fingers so that it does not obstruct the dowsing.

You will need to ascertain which is a 'yes' and which a 'no' response. Some people find that the pendulum swings in one direction for 'yes' and at right angles to that axis for 'no', while others have a backwards and forwards swing for one reply, and a circular motion for the other. A 'wobble' of the pendulum can indicate a 'maybe' or that it is not appropriate to dowse at that time, or that the wrong question is being asked. In which case, ask if it is appropriate, and if the answer is 'yes', check that you are framing the question in the correct way. If the pendulum stops completely it is usually inappropriate to ask at that time.

You can ascertain your particular pendulum response by holding the pendulum over your knee and asking: "Is my name [correct name]?" The direction that the pendulum swings will indicate 'yes'. Check by asking: "Is my name [incorrect name]?" to establish 'no'. Or, you can program in 'yes' and 'no' by swinging the pendulum in a particular direction a few times, saying as you do: "This is yes" and swinging it in a different direction to program in "no".

Once you have established yes or no, hold the

pendulum over each chakra in turn and ask to be shown whether the chakra is open or closed, whether it is balanced or in need of attention. You will soon learn to recognize the response.

To dowse the best crystal for you

To ascertain which crystal will be most beneficial for you or for your purpose, hold the pendulum in your most receptive hand. Put the forefinger of your other hand on the chakra, condition or issue in the directory. Slowly run your finger along the list of possible crystals, noting whether you get a 'yes' or 'no' response. Check the whole list to see which 'yes' response is strongest as there may well be two or three that would be appropriate, or you may need to use several crystals in combination. Another way to do this, if you have several of the crystals available, is to touch each crystal in turn, again noting the 'yes' or 'no' response – open your palm chakras before doing so (see page 60).

If you get a 'no' response when checking out a condition or chakra, open your palm chakras, touch each of the capital letters in turn dowsing until you receive a 'yes', then run your finger down the entries until you get a 'yes'. This may well reveal something that underlies the apparent issue or blockage. If you get no response at all, it may be that you need to remove yourself from a geopathically stressed place, or that the question should be asked at another time.

Alternatively, if you have a selection of crystals, open

the palm chakras in your hands and allow your hands to simply find the right crystal, without thinking about it, which will feel tingly or may jump out of your hands as you pick it up.

Purifying, Re-energizing and Focusing Your Crystals

Purifying your crystal

As crystals hold the energetic charge of everyone who comes into contact with them and rapidly absorb emanations from their surroundings as well as your personal energies they need regular purifying. It is sensible to cleanse and re-energize a crystal every time it is used. The method employed will depend on the type of crystal. Soft and friable crystals, for instance, and those that are attached to a base may be damaged by water, and soft stones such as Selenite will dissolve. These are best purified by a 'dry' process such as brown rice, sounds, smudging or sun or moonlight, but sturdier crystals benefit from being placed under running water or in the sea. *Remember, all crystals benefit from regular cleansing, even those that may be stated never to need cleansing such as Shungite, which responds well to crystal clearing essences or immersing in brown rice or directly into the earth. Re-energize in the light of the sun or with Clear2Light.*

Methods:

Running water

Hold your crystals under a running tap, or pour bottled water over them, or place in them a stream or the ocean to draw off negative energy (use a bag to hold small crystals). You can also immerse appropriate crystals in a bowl of water into which a handful of sea salt or rock salt has been added. (Salt is best avoided if the crystal is layered or friable.) Dry the crystal carefully afterwards and place in the sun to re-energize or use a proprietary crystal essence.

Returning to the earth

You will need to dowse to establish the length of time a crystal needs to return to the earth in order to cleanse and recharge as the period will differ with each crystal. If you do not have a garden, a flowerpot filled with soil or sand can be used instead and is very handy for crystals that require a daily cleanse and regrounding. If you bury crystals to cleanse them, remember to mark the spot.

Rice or salt

Brown rice seems to have a special affinity with crystals that have been subjected to EMF pollution, rapidly drawing it off. Salt also works but can be damaging to layered or friable crystals. Place your crystal in a bowl of brown rice or salt (unless layered or friable) and leave overnight for the negative energies to be absorbed. Brush the salt off carefully and make sure that it has been removed from any niches or cracks in the crystal as otherwise it will absorb water in the future and could cause splintering. Place the crystals in the sun to re-energize if appropriate or use a proprietary crystal essence. Compost or discard the rice, do not eat.

Smudging

Sage, sweetgrass or joss sticks are excellent for smudging as they quickly remove negative energies. Light the smudge stick and pass it over the crystal if it is large, or hold the crystal in your hand in the smoke if it is small. It is traditional to fan the smoke gently with a feather but this is not essential.

Visualizing light

Hold your crystal in your hands and visualize a column of bright white light coming down and covering the crystal, absorbing anything negative it may have picked up and restoring the pure energy once more. If you find visualization difficult, you can use the light of a candle. Crystals also respond well to being placed in sun or moonlight to cleanse and recharge.

Sound

A Tibetan bowl, tingshas or tuning forks can all cleanse crystal energy. Simply sound over the crystal and then place it in the sun to re-energize.

Crystal clearing essences

Clearing essences are ideal as they prepare a crystal for use whenever you need it, or cleanse it after use so that it can immediately be used again. A number of crystal clearing essences are available from flower essence suppliers, crystal shops and the Internet (see Resources). Personally I never move far without Clear2Light, a crystal and space clearing essence that also re-energizes the crystal. You can either drop the essence directly on to the crystal, gently rubbing it over the crystal with your finger, or put a few drops into clean spring water in an atomiser or spray bottle and gently mist the crystal.

Re-energizing your Crystal

Crystals can be placed on a Quartz cluster or on a large Carnelian to re-energize them. Or, you can use a proprietary crystal recharger (Petaltone and the Crystal Balance Company make excellent ones, see Resources) but the light of the sun is an excellent natural energizer. Red and yellow crystals particularly enjoy being placed in the sun, and white and pale-coloured crystals respond well to the moon. Be aware that sunlight focused through a crystal can be a fire hazard and delicate crystals will lose their colour quickly if left exposed to light. Some brown crystals such as Smoky Quartz respond to being placed on or in the earth to recharge. If you bury a crystal, remember to mark its position clearly.

Focusing and activating your crystal

Crystals work best when their energy is harnessed and focused with intent towards the task at hand as this activates them. By taking the time to attune a crystal to your own unique frequency, you enhance its vibratory effect and amplify its healing power. Once your crystal has been purified and re-energized, sit quietly holding the crystal in your hands for a few minutes until you feel in tune with it. Picture it surrounded by light and love. State that the crystal is dedicated to the highest good of all who use it. Then state very clearly your intention for the crystal – that it will balance or open your chakras, for instance, or that it will transmute negative energy. If it is intended for a specific purpose such as healing a particular chakra or issue, state that also. Repeat the intention several times to anchor it into the crystal.

Using Your Crystals

Crystals can be laid directly on the chakras (see page 21), or placed at a distance around the body (see figure of eight page 120). To raise kundalini, they can be laid along the spine or used as directed (see page 158). Many of the directory entries indicate a chakra link through which a chakra can be activated and purified, or a condition healed. You can dowse for or intuit the most appropriate of the crystals listed. Most crystals can be placed over clothing on the chakra, or over organs or the site of disease, and left in place for fifteen to twenty minutes or so. Crystals can also be taped in place, or worn for much longer periods for healing, activation or rebalancing; or they can be placed beneath your mattress.

If your crystal has a point, place it point towards yourself, or point down if placed on your body, to draw in healing or re-energizing properties down into your body. Place it point up to draw Qi or kundalini energy from the base of the spine. Place it point out, or point down below your feet to draw off toxic residues or emotional debris. When you have placed the stones, close your eyes and breathe gently and evenly, and allow yourself to relax and feel the energy of the crystal radiating out through your whole being. Hold the intention that the stones will work for you.

You can also apply crystal essences (see pages 180–184). These essences convey crystal vibes to the body at a subtle level, repatterning your cells and the spaces in between to optimum.

Working with a variety of types and colours of crystals helps you to find which ones best suit your own particular energy frequency – you don't have to buy them all. Use the colour photographs in my books or on crystal websites to tune into the stones and dowse for those which are right for you. I particularly recommend www.exquisitecrystals.com as John Jnr. took the excellent photographs in *101 Power Crystals* and *Crystals and Sacred Sites*, and www.angeladditions.co.uk which is my daughter's website. You could also use the stunning photographs from my *Crystal Wisdom Oracle*.

Crystal massage

An alternative to laying crystals on the chakras or over an organ is to use one to massage the site. Tumbled stones and wands with rounded ends are most suitable but you can use crystals with points – in which case start a little way off the body and work down towards it before gently massaging the spot so that you ascertain the appropriate pressure to apply.

You can also spiral crystals out from a chakra to cleanse it and then back in again to recharge it. Don't worry too much about the direction of the spiral. Let your hand follow the crystal's instructions. It may be necessary to cleanse the crystal before reversing the spin back in, however.

How long should I use a crystal?

A pendulum can be used to establish how long a crystal should be left in place. This is particularly useful if you are placing the crystal at a chakra or over an organ, but it can also be helpful if you are wearing a crystal and need to know whether or not to wear it at night – in which case you will get a 'yes' or 'no' answer to the question: "Should I remove this crystal at night?" To establish timing, use an arc on which you have marked five-minute or one-hour or one-day intervals (ask in advance whether the period should be checked in minutes, hours or days). Hold the hand with the pendulum over the centre of the arc and ask that the pendulum will go towards the correct period (see illustration).

Healing challenge

Occasionally a crystal will trigger a 'healing challenge' when the 'symptoms' appear to get worse rather than better and flu-like symptoms may occur. This is an indication of physical, emotional or mental toxins leaving the body and is all part of the process. It occurs particularly in stress-related or chronic conditions, or when a blocked chakra or energy body is released. It can be soothed and facilitated by crystals such as Smoky Elestial Quartz, Eye of the Storm, Spirit Quartz or Quantum Quattro and by drinking plenty of water (Shungite-infused water is ideal). If a healing challenge occurs use these stones for a few days until the symptoms dissipate and then return to the crystals you were using – having dowsed or intuited if they are still appropriate.

Crystal Essences

Crystal essences are an excellent way to use the healing power of crystals, and several crystals can be combined provided you dowse to check compatibility. The essence can be gently rubbed on the skin over a chakra. Essences can also be added to a glass of water and sipped, or taken from a dropper bottle, or sprayed around the aura. Crystal essences are made by transferring the subtle energies and minute concentrations of the mineral constituents of the crystal into water, which then stores the vibrations and transfers them to the chakras, physical or subtle bodies in exactly the same way that a homoeopathic essence works. The essence is bottled and a preservative – brandy, vodka or cider vinegar – added. If the essence is to be taken by those for whom alcohol is inappropriate, cider vinegar can be used as a preservative or the essence rubbed on the skin. (See Resources for purpose-made highly effective essences.)

Caution: Some stones contain trace minerals that are toxic (see the list in Contraindications) and essences from these stones need to be made by an indirect method that transfers the vibrations without transferring any of the toxic material from the stone (see page 241). If in doubt, make the essence by the indirect method, which is also suitable for fragile or layered stones. Always wash your hands after handling one of these stones and use in a tumbled version wherever possible.

Making a crystal essence

You will need the appropriate crystal, which has been cleansed and purified (see pages 173–176), one or two clean glass bowls, spring water and a suitable bottle in which to keep the essence (coloured glass is preferable to clear as it preserves the vibrations better). Essences can be made by the direct or indirect method. The indirect method is suitable for friable, layered or clustered crystals as well as those that may have a degree of toxicity. Spring water should be used rather than tap water that has chlorine, fluoride and aluminium added to it. Water from a spring with healing properties is particularly effective.

Direct method

Place enough spring water in a glass bowl to just cover the crystal. Stand the bowl in sunlight for several hours. (If the bowl is left outside, cover with a glass lid or cling film to prevent insects falling into it.) If appropriate, the bowl can also be left overnight in moonlight.

Indirect method

If the crystal is toxic or fragile (see Contraindications page 241) place the crystal in a small glass bowl and stand the bowl within a large bowl that has sufficient spring water to raise the level above the crystal in the inner bowl. Stand the bowl in sunlight for several hours. (If the bowl is left outside, cover with a glass lid or cling film.) If appropriate, the bowl can also be left overnight in moonlight.

Bottling and preserving

If the essence is not to be used within a day or two, top up with two-thirds brandy, vodka, white rum or cider vinegar to one-third essence, otherwise the essence will become musty. This makes a 'mother tincture' that can be further diluted. To make a small dosage bottle, add seven drops of the mother essence to a dosage bottle containing two-thirds brandy and one-third water. If a spray bottle is being made, add seven drops of mother essence to pure water if using immediately. For prolonged use, vodka or white rum makes a useful preservative as they have no smell.

Using a crystal essence

For short-term use, an essence can be sipped every few minutes or rubbed on the appropriate chakra. Hold the water in your mouth for a few moments. Essences can also be applied to the skin, either at the wrist or over the site of a problem, or added to bath water. If a spray bottle is made, spray all around the aura and at the site of particular chakras remembering that these can extend for several feet out from the physical body or room. This is particularly effective for clearing negative energies.

Making Shungite water

To become biologically active, water needs to have Shungite immersed in it for at least 48 hours. However, once the first batch has been made, you can simply refill the filter jug every time you use some of the water so that it is constantly replenished. Wash the jug and the bag of Shungite at least once a week depending on how much water you have used (you can store the activated water and return it to the jug). Place the Shungite in the sun for a few hours to recharge or use a proprietary crystal recharging essence. I find raw Shungite more effective than the silvery tumbles, but, no matter how often the non-vitreous type of Shungite has been washed, it does tend to leave a very fine suspension of black particles in the water. I have drunk this for several years now without any ill effects and, indeed, I believe it to have contributed greatly to my overall well-being.

Making the water

You will need:

2-litre filter jug
Fine mesh 2″ bag of raw Shungite (10–100gm)

Place the mesh bag of Shungite in the base of the filter jug (if using tap water you can also use a commercial filter if the jug is provided with one). Pour water into the jug until it is full. Stand it aside for 48 hours. Then top up the water each time it is used. Cleanse the Shungite frequently under running water and re-energize in the sun or fresh air.

Case Histories

Maybe an example or two will help here. Under current EU regulations, I cannot claim that a crystal 'cures' but I am allowed to share anecdotal experiences of their use with you.

Opening the psychic gateways

Many workshop participants either develop a migraine-type headache during the workshop, or arrive complaining that they've had one for days, weeks or even years – usually since they began their spiritual seeking. I most often attribute this to blocked psychic energy at the third eye (brow) chakra. But it can also be a blocked alta major chakra, although if the tension is tightest around the back of the head it links to the past life chakras as well.

My tried and tested remedy for the third eye chakra headache is a Bytownite (Yellow Labradorite), Rhomboid Blue Selenite, Optical Calcite or Apophyllite crystal soaked in Petaltone Greenaway or Leaf 1 essence. Placed on the chakra, it clears any blockage almost instantaneously, the headache disappears, and inner sight is released. If the blockage is at a higher frequency,

Diaspore may be needed. Such blockages are often created by restrictions or strictures to silence placed on psychic sight in other lives so a Banded Agate may also help. This is particularly so where the person has been working under the guidance of a guru. Some work on the past life chakras may also be needed.

If the alta major is blocked, placing a Blue Moonstone or one of the other psychic gateway releasing crystals in the hollow at the back of the skull where the spine begins is usually sufficient to clear the pathways and reconnect this complex chakra inside the skull, restoring it to equilibrium. It may, however, need another crystal such as Preseli Bluestone on the third eye or the soma chakra to complete and anchor the rebalancing.

If the blockage is intractable, as in the case of Tony, then a more intensive approach may be needed. Tony "desperately wanted to be able to see" but he was also afraid of the consequences – which we traced to a past life scenario that had to be cleared with regression therapy first. Once the past life had been reframed, placing Auralite 23 around his head with Apophyllite on the third eye, Diaspore on the soma chakra and Blue Moonstone at the base of the skull quickly opened up his metaphysical abilities. He began training as a psychic and is now doing that work fulltime.

The kundalini fountain

I had a new stone, Triplite, on trial and took it to a workshop. I had already found that it fired up creativity, but was interested to know what its effect would be on the chakras. Mary felt very blocked both in her inner life and her outer. She said she could not express who she was nor access her talents. She volunteered to try the new stone. We laid small pieces of Triplite on Mary's chakras, starting at the base and moving towards the head, above which Petalite had been placed on the stellar gateway. Energy began to shoot upwards, rippling through her body, and she became light-headed and spacy. Putting a piece of the Triplite matrix (tiny specks of Triplite in a rock base) below her feet on the Gaia gateway anchored the energy. Triplite is a very high-energy stone and a piece of Smoky Quartz on the earth star was not sufficient. The flow moved more gently but still dynamically through the chakras, rising to the stellar gateway and then falling back down through her energy bodies to the Gaia gateway where it began to move upwards once more. Mary reported feeling much more energized and connected. In a later communication she told me that her life had taken a sudden turn for the better after the workshop. She'd found a job she really liked, her health had improved, and she had begun to write in her spare time. At the time I wasn't thinking in terms of kundalini flow but with hindsight it had looked, with a psychic eye, exactly like a kundalini fountain finding its proper channel through which to flow and move her life forward.

Balancing the yogic effect

Freya had begun an introductory course of kundalini yoga which worked on each of the chakras in turn. She missed a week of the course, that covering the solar plexus chakra. She had had great sadness in her life which was locked into that chakra, although she did not realize that when she began the course. She returned to the course, seemingly progressing well but did not fill in the missing step. She began to suffer from extreme insomnia. She would have great difficulty falling asleep, only to awake with a start a few minutes later, and that went on throughout the night. She developed chronic back problems just over the heart chakra and along to under her left arm, which she could not lift. It made the yoga difficult but she persevered. She did not initially link her symptoms to the yoga or blocked chakras as she had experienced a similar problem several times before. Halfway through the advanced course she had to put it on hold as her partner became seriously ill and needed her constant support. By the time he had recovered, she was extremely depleted. She was still not sleeping, had no energy and developed a severe kidney infection, and the back problem remained despite chiropractic treatment. Kidneys are linked to fear and she had had a very real fear that her partner would die. But kidneys are also linked to the sacral and spleen chakras. Dowsing revealed that the sacral chakra was locked shut, and the spleen was wide open and spinning madly. Her heart chakra flow was distressed as a result.

Greenish-yellow Zincite taped over the kidneys helped the infection to ease and the fear to be gently released, a process that was supported by Bloodstone on her higher heart chakra. Her sacral chakra was treated with Jade to release the blockage and then Citrine to restore the energy. Her spleen chakra spin was restored to normal and protected with Green Aventurine. Her heart was then treated with a series of crystals: Rose Quartz to bring it back into equilibrium and fill it with love, Tugtupite to activate the heart seed and Pink Petalite to open it to a higher resonance. Kundalini Quartz at the base of her spine and Serpentine above her head equalised the kundalini flow through the whole chakra system. She wore an Eye of the Storm on a long chain to maintain her stability and give her a peaceful core. Her kidney infection healed, her back problem eased, and she was able to return to her yoga class to complete the process of kundalini activation.

Using This Directory

In this directory you will first find an alphabetical list of the chakras and their balancing crystals, followed by a list of the subtle bodies and their healing crystals. The final part of the directory is an A–Z list of symptoms that are associated with chakra imbalances and kundalini awakening. In addition, the directory has crystals for the organs, glands and systems of the body governed by the chakras as well as those for mitigating the side effects of kundalini rise. Most entries have several crystals listed that would be beneficial, although a few have only one. There is a choice because everyone is subtly different and deeper causes may underlie a symptom. Crystals heal holistically – that is to say they work at a causal level on the whole person. What works for you will not necessarily work for your friend because you will have different causes for your dis-ease or chakra blockage, and you will have different body types, ancestral factors or chakra blockages. Many of the entries also have a chakra or chakras associated with them. This means that a condition can be treated, or a chakra restored to optimum functioning, through putting appropriate stones on the appropriate chakra and leaving in place for fifteen to twenty minutes or so.

To identify the right crystal, check out your chakras, symptom, condition or issue and dowse or intuit which crystal is appropriate. There may be more than one. In which case ask, "Which crystal will be the most beneficial at this time?" If you have several blockages or issues, you may well find that one crystal is beneficial for all. This will be the crystal for you. It could be that you already own the crystal, having been instinctively drawn to it. But you may be left with a choice of several crystals, in which case turn to page 166 to learn how to identify the one that will be of greatest benefit to you, although many crystals work well in combination. Occasionally certain crystals are contraindicated and you will find these listed in the directory under Contraindications (page 241).

Many problems arise in the first instance from blocked chakras or repressed emotions – which will in turn be stored in the appropriate chakra. So, to find the source of a problem, check out the chakra physiology and effect of blockages. If you have endocrine problems, for instance, you may need to check that the alta major chakra is functioning optimally. If your eyes are troubling you, as well as looking deeply into what you do not wish to see, or what you are blocking out from your sight, you will also need to ascertain if the alta major or third eye is functioning optimally. Placing crystals on the appropriate chakra will assist in healing the core issue. The entries have the appropriate chakras alongside.

You can also apply crystal essences to the chakras or to the subtle energy bodies (see pages 180–184). These essences convey crystal vibes to the body at a subtle level and are particularly effective for assimilating high vibrational downloads and making soul shifts.

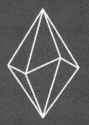

Part II

A – Z Directory of
Crystal Solutions

The Chakras and Their Activation Crystals

Alta Major chakra: Afghanite, African Jade (Budd Stone), Anandalite, Andara Glass, Angelinite, Angel's Wing Calcite, Apatite, Auralite 23, Aurichalcite, Azeztulite, Black Moonstone, Blue Moonstone, Brandenberg Amethyst, Crystal Cap Amethyst, Diaspore (Zultanite), Emerald, Ethiopian Opal, Eye of the Storm (Judy's Jasper), Fire and Ice Quartz, Fluorapatite, Garnet in Pyroxene, Graphic Smoky Quartz, Green Ridge Quartz, Golden Healer, Golden Herkimer Diamond, Holly Agate, Hungarian Quartz, Petalite, Phenacite, Preseli Bluestone, Rainbow Covellite, Rainbow Mayanite, Red Agate, Red Amethyst, Rosophia. Place at base of skull.

> **balance and align:** Anandalite, Brandenberg Amethyst, Crystal Cap Amethyst; Green Ridge Quartz, Preseli Bluestone on soma chakra with Angel's Wing Calcite or Herkimer Diamond on base of skull

> **spin too rapid/stuck open:** African Jade (Budd Stone), Auralite 23, Black Moonstone, Calcite, Eye of the

---

Unless otherwise directed, apply crystal over chakras, organ or site of symptom, wear as jewellery, bathe with or use as crystal essence.

Storm, Flint, Golden Healer, Graphic Smoky Quartz

spin too sluggish/stuck closed: Blue Moonstone, Diaspore, Ethiopian Opal, Herkimer Diamond, Quartz, Red Agate

Base chakra: Amber, Azurite, Bastnasite, Black Obsidian, Black Opal, Black Tourmaline, Bloodstone, Candle Quartz, Carnelian, Chinese Red Quartz, Chrysocolla, Cinnabar Jasper, Citrine, Clinohumite, Cuprite, Dragon Stone, Eye of the Storm (Judy's Jasper), Fire Agate, Fulgarite, Gabbro, Garnet, Golden Topaz, Harlequin Quartz (Hematite in Quartz), Hematite, Kambaba Jasper, Keyiapo, Limonite, Obsidian, Pink Tourmaline, Poppy Jasper, Realgar and Orpiment, Red Amethyst, Red Calcite, Red Jasper, Red Zincite, Ruby, Serpentine, Serpentine in Obsidian, Shungite, Smoky Quartz, Sonora Sunrise, Spinel, Stromatolite, Tangerose, Triplite, Zircon. *Chakra:* Place at perineum or base of spine

> **balance and align:** Anandalite, Celestobarite, Green Ridge Quartz, Hematite Quartz, Red Calcite, Red Coral, Ruby, Shiva Lingam
>
> **spin too rapid/stuck open:** Agate, Green Ridge Quartz, Mahogany Obsidian, Pink Tourmaline, Smoky Quartz, Triplite matrix
>
> **spin too sluggish/stuck closed:** Fire Agate, Hematite, Kundalini Quartz, Red Calcite, Serpentine, Sonora Sunrise, Triplite

---

Unless otherwise directed, apply crystal over chakras, organ or site of symptom, wear as jewellery, bathe with or use as crystal essence.

Causal Vortex chakra: Ajoite, Apatite, Azeztulite, Banded White Agate, Black or Blue Moonstone, Blue Kyanite, Brandenberg Amethyst, Chrysotile, Cobalto Calcite, Cryolite, Crystalline Blue Kyanite, Diamond, Diaspore (Zultanite), Fluorapatite, Herderite, Petalite, Phenacite, Rainbow Moonstone, Scolecite, Sugilite, Tanzanite

> **balance and align:** Anandalite, Brandenberg Amethyst, Chrysotile, Crystalline Blue Kyanite, Fluorapatite, Phenacite, Scolecite, Smoky Elestial Quartz
>
> **spin too rapid/stuck open:** Black Moonstone, Cobalto Calcite, Diaspore, Scolecite with Natrolite
>
> **spin too sluggish/stuck closed:** Ajoite, Blue Moonstone, Herderite, Petalite, Tanzanite

Crown chakra: Afghanite, Amethyst, Amphibole Quartz, Angelite, Angel's Wing Calcite, Arfvedsonite, Auralite 23, Brandenberg Amethyst, Brookite, Celestial Quartz, Citrine, Clear Tourmaline, Diaspore (Zultanite), Golden Beryl, Golden Healer, Green Ridge Quartz, Herderite, Heulandite, Larimar, Lepidolite, Moldavite, Natrolite, Novaculite, Petalite, Phenacite, Purple Jasper, Purple Sapphire, Quartz, Rosophia, Satyamani and Satyaloka Quartz, Scolecite, Selenite, Serpentine, Sugilite, Titanite (Sphene), Trigonic, White Calcite, White Topaz. *Chakra:* crown, top of head

> **balance and align:** Amethyst, Anandalite, Auralite 23,

Brandenberg Amethyst, Phenacite, Selenite, Sugilite

spin too rapid/stuck open: Amethyst, Amphibole Quartz, Larimar, Petalite, Serpentine, White Calcite

spin too sluggish/stuck closed: Moldavite, Phenacite, Rosophia, Selenite

Dantien chakra: Amber, Carnelian, Chinese Red Quartz, Empowerite, Eye of the Storm, Fire Agate, Fire Opal, Green Ridge Quartz, Golden Herkimer, Hematite, Hematoid Calcite, Kambaba Jasper, Madagascan Red Celestial Quartz, Moonstone, Orange River Quartz, Peanut Wood, Polychrome Jasper, Poppy Jasper, Red Amethyst, Red Jasper, Rhodozite, Rose or Ruby Aura Quartz, Rosophia, Stromatolite, Topaz

>**balance and align:** Empowerite, Eye of the Storm, Green Ridge Quartz, Poppy Jasper
>
>**spin too rapid/stuck open:** Peanut Wood, Polychrome Jasper, Stromatolite
>
>**spin too sluggish/stuck closed:** Fire Agate, Fire Opal, Hematite, Madagascan Red Celestial Quartz, Poppy Jasper, Red Jasper

Earth Star chakra: Agnitite™, Boji Stone, Brown Jasper, Celestobarite, Champagne Aura Quartz, Cuprite, Fire Agate, Flint, Galena (wash hands after use, make essence by indirect method), Golden Herkimer, Graphic Smoky Quartz, Hematite, Lemurian Jade, Limonite, Madagascan Red Celestial Quartz, Mahogany Obsidian,

Unless otherwise directed, apply crystal over chakras, organ or site of symptom, wear as jewellery, bathe with or use as crystal essence.

Proustite, Red Amethyst, Rhodonite, Rhodozite, Rosophia, Smoky Elestial Quartz, Smoky Quartz, Thunder Egg, Tourmaline. Place below feet.

balance and align: Blue Flint, Brown-flash Anandalite, Green Ridge Quartz, Hematite, Smoky Elestial Quartz

spin too rapid/stuck open: Flint, Graphic Smoky Quartz, Green Ridge Quartz, Smoky Quartz

spin too sluggish/stuck closed: Golden Herkimer, Hematite, Red Amethyst, Rhodozite, Thunder Egg

Gaia Gateway chakra: Apache Tear, Basalt, Basanite, Black Actinolite, Black Calcite, Black Flint, Black Kyanite, Black Obsidian, Black Petalite, Black Spinel, Black Spot Herkimer Diamond, Day and Night Quartz, Fire and Ice, Jet, Master Shamanite, Mohawkite, Morion, Naturally Dark Smoky Quartz (not irradiated), Nebula Stone, Nirvana Quartz, Nuummite, Petalite, Preseli Bluestone, Sardonyx, Shungite, Smoky Elestial Quartz, Snowflake Obsidian, Specular Hematite, Spider Web Obsidian, Stromatolite, Tektite, Tibetan Black Spot Quartz, Tourmalinated Quartz, Verdelite. *Chakra:* below feet and/or on stellar gateway

balance and align: Black Flint, Day and Night Quartz, Fire and Ice, Master Shamanite, Morion, Shungite, Tourmalinated Quartz, Verdelite

spin too rapid/stuck open: Apache Tear, Basalt, Black Flint, Black Kyanite, Master Shamanite, Sardonyx,

Shungite

spin too sluggish/stuck closed: Black Spot Herkimer Diamond, Nirvana Quartz, Preseli Bluestone, Shungite, Specular Hematite, Tektite, Tibetan Black Spot Quartz

Heart chakra: Apophyllite, Aventurine, Chrysocolla, Chrysoprase, Cobalto Calcite, Danburite, Eudialyte, Gaia Stone, Green Jasper, Green Quartz, Green Sapphire, Green Siberian Quartz, Green Tourmaline, Hematite Quartz, Herkimer Diamond, Jade, Jadeite, Kunzite, Lavender Quartz, Lepidolite, Malachite, Morganite, Muscovite, Pink Danburite, Pink Petalite, Pink Tourmaline, Pyroxmangite, Red Calcite, Rhodochrosite, Rhodonite, Rhodozaz, Rose Quartz, Rubellite Tourmaline, Ruby, Ruby Lavender Quartz, Tugtupite, Variscite, Watermelon Tourmaline

   balance and align: Anandalite, Cobalto Calcite, Kunzite, Mangano Calcite, Ruby Lavender Quartz, Watermelon Tourmaline

   clear heart chakra attachments: Banded Agate, Mangano Calcite

   open the three-chambered heart: Danburite, Lemurian Aquitane Calcite, Mangano Calcite, Pink Petalite, Pink Tourmaline, Rosophia, Tugtupite

   spin too rapid/stuck open: Green Tourmaline, Mangano Calcite, Quartz, Rose Quartz, Tugtupite

   spin too sluggish/stuck closed: Calcite, Chohua

Unless otherwise directed, apply crystal over chakras, organ or site of symptom, wear as jewellery, bathe with or use as crystal essence.

Jasper, Danburite, Erythrite, Honey Calcite, Lemurian Jade, Pink Lemurian Seed, Red Calcite, Rhodozaz, Rose Quartz, Strawberry Quartz, Tugtupite

Heart Seed chakra: Ajo Blue Calcite, Ajoite, Azeztulite, Brandenberg Amethyst, Coral, Danburite, Dianite, Fire Opal, Golden Healer, Green Ridge Quartz, Khutnohorite, Lemurian Calcite, Lilac Quartz, Macedonian Opal, Mangano Calcite, Merkabite Calcite, Pink Opal, Pyroxmangite, Rhodozaz, Roselite, Rosophia, Ruby Lavender Quartz, Scolecite, Spirit Quartz, Tugtupite, Violane. Place at base of breastbone.

> **balance and align:** Danburite, Golden Healer, Golden Herkimer, Khutnohorite, Merkabite Calcite
> **spin too rapid/stuck open:** Ajo Blue Calcite, Khutnohorite, Macedonian Opal
> **spin too sluggish/stuck closed:** Fire Opal, Rhodozaz, Rosophia, Spirit Quartz

Higher Heart chakra: Ajo Blue Calcite, Amazonite, Anandalite (Aurora Quartz), Aqua Aura Quartz, Azeztulite, Bloodstone, Celestite, Danburite, Dioptase, Dream Quartz, Eye of the Storm, Fire and Ice Quartz, Gaia Stone, Green Siberian Quartz, Khutnohorite, Kunzite, Lavender Quartz, Lazurine, Lilac Quartz, Macedonian Opal, Mangano Calcite, Muscovite, Nirvana Quartz, Phenacite, Pink Crackle Quartz, Pink or Lilac Danburite, Pink Lazurine, Pink Petalite, Pyroxmangite,

Unless otherwise directed, apply crystal over chakras, organ or site of symptom, wear as jewellery, bathe with or use as crystal essence.

Quantum Quattro, Que Sera, Rainbow Mayanite, Raspberry Aura Quartz, Rhodozaz, Rose Elestial Quartz, Roselite, Rose Opal, Rose Quartz, Rosophia, Ruby Aura Quartz, Ruby Lavender Quartz™, Spirit Quartz, Strawberry Lemurian, Strawberry Quartz, Tangerose, Tugtupite, Turquoise. *Chakra:* higher heart

> **balance and align:** Bloodstone, Eye of the Storm, Quantum Quattro, Que Sera, Tangerose
>
> **spin too rapid/stuck open:** Eye of the Storm, Mangano Calcite, Pink Petalite, Rose Elestial Quartz, Turquoise
>
> **spin too sluggish/stuck closed:** Quantum Quattro, Que Sera, Ruby Aura Quartz, Strawberry Lemurian

Knee chakras: Aragonite, Azurite, Blue Lace Agate, Boji Stone, Cathedral Quartz, Dinosaur Bone, Flint, Hematite, Magnetite, Merlinite, Peanut Wood, Petrified Wood, Preseli Bluestone, Shungite with Selenite, Sodalite, Spider Web Obsidian, Stromatolite

> **balance and align:** Aragonite, Magnetite, Mohawkite, Polychrome Jasper, Preseli Bluestone with chalk
>
> **spin too rapid/stuck open:** Flint, Hematite, Mohawkite, Polychrome Jasper, Smoky Quartz
>
> **spin too sluggish/stuck closed:** Fire Opal, Harlequin Quartz, Hematite Quartz

Palm chakras: Flint, Quartz, Spangolite. *Chakra:* throat, third eye, soma, crown

---

Unless otherwise directed, apply crystal over chakras, organ or site of symptom, wear as jewellery, bathe with or use as crystal essence.

balance and align: Anandalite, Quartz

spin too rapid/stuck open: Flint, Granite, Hematite

spin too sluggish/stuck open: Quartz, Spangolite

Note: any crystal will open the palm chakras

Past Life chakras: Ammolite, Astraline, Black Moonstone, Blizzard Stone, Brandenberg Amethyst, Catlinite, Chrysotile, Chrysotile in Serpentine, Coprolite, Cuprite with Chrysocolla, Dinosaur Bone, Dumortierite, Ethiopian Opal, Fire and Ice, Flint, Keyiapo, Larvikite, Lemurian Aquatine Calcite, Madagascar Quartz, Mystic Merlinite, Oceanite (Blue Onyx), Peanut Wood, Petrified Wood, Preseli Bluestone, Rainbow Mayanite, Rainbow Moonstone, Reinerite, Rhodozite, Rhyolite, Scheelite, Serpentine in Obsidian, Shiva Lingam, Smoky Amethyst, Tangerose, Tantalite, Titanite, Variscite, Violane (Blue Dioptase), Voegesite, Wind Fossil Agate

balance and align: Dumortierite, Picasso Jasper, Rainbow Mayanite, Tangerose, Titanite, Violane (Blue Dioptase)

spin too rapid/stuck open: Black Moonstone, Coprolite, Flint, Petrified Wood, Preseli Bluestone, Scheelite, Sea Sediment Jasper, Tantalite

spin too sluggish/stuck closed: Blizzard Stone, Dragon Stone, Dumortierite, Garnet in Quartz, Rhodozite, Serpentine in Obsidian, Tantalite

Sacral chakra: Amber, Amphibole, Bastnasite, Black

Opal, Blue-green Fluorite, Blue-green Turquoise, Blue Jasper, Bumble Bee Jasper, Carnelian, Chinese Red Quartz, Citrine, Clinohumite, Golden and iron-coated Green Ridge Quartz, Golden Healer Quartz, Keyiapo, Limonite, Mahogany Obsidian, Orange Calcite, Orange Carnelian, Orange Kyanite, Orange Zincite, Realgar and Orpiment, Red Amethyst, Red Jasper, Red/Orange Zincite, Tangerose, Topaz, Triplite, Vanadinite. *Chakra:* sacral/navel

> **balance and align:** Anandalite, Celestobarite, Golden Healer Quartz, Green Ridge Quartz
>
> **spin too rapid/stuck open:** Amber, Black Opal, Blue-green Fluorite, Blue-green Turquoise
>
> **spin too sluggish/stuck closed:** Carnelian, Orange Zincite, Topaz, Triplite

Solar Plexus chakra: Calcite, Citrine, Citrine Herkimer, Golden Azeztulite, Golden Beryl, Golden Calcite, Golden Coracalcite, Golden Danburite, Golden Enhydro, Golden Healer, Golden Labradorite (Bytownite), Green Chrysoprase, Green Prehnite, Green Ridge Quartz, Jasper, Libyan Glass Tektite, Light Green Hiddenite, Malachite (use as polished stone, make essence by indirect method), Obsidian, Rainbow Obsidian, Rhodochrosite, Rhodozite, Smoky Quartz, Sunstone, Tangerine Aura Quartz, Tangerine Dream Lemurian Seed, Tiger's Eye, Yellow Tourmaline, Yellow Zincite

> **balance and align:** Anandalite, Citrine, Lemurian

Seed

spin too rapid/stuck open: Calcite, Light Green Hiddenite, Malachite, Rainbow Obsidian, Smoky Quartz

spin too sluggish/stuck closed: Golden Calcite, Golden Danburite, Tangerine Aura Quartz, Yellow Labradorite (Bytownite)

Soma chakra: Afghanite, Amechlorite, Angelinite, Angel's Wing Calcite, Astraline, Auralite 23, Azeztulite, Banded Agate, Brandenberg Amethyst, Champagne Aura Quartz, Crystal Cap Amethyst, Diaspore (Zultanite), Faden Quartz, Fire and Ice, Holly Agate, Ilmenite, Isis Calcite, Lemurian Aquatine Calcite, Merkabite Calcite, Natrolite, Nuummite, Owyhee Blue Opal, Pentagonite, Petalite, Phantom Calcite, Phenacite on Fluorite, Preseli Bluestone, Red Amethyst, Sacred Scribe, Satyaloka and Satyamani Quartz, Scolecite, Sedona Stone, Shaman Quartz, Stellar Beam Calcite, Trigonic Quartz, Violane, Z-stone. *Chakra:* soma, mid-hairline

balance and align: Bytownite, Diaspore, Stellar Beam Calcite, Violane

spin too rapid/stuck open: Isis Calcite, Pinky-beige Ussingite, Sedona Stone, Shaman Quartz, White Banded Agate

spin too sluggish/stuck closed: Banded Agate, Diaspore, Nuummite, Preseli Bluestone

---

Unless otherwise directed, apply crystal over chakras, organ or site of symptom, wear as jewellery, bathe with or use as crystal essence.

Soul Star chakra: Afghanite, Ajoite, Amethyst Elestial, Amphibole, Anandalite, Angel's Wing Calcite, Apophyllite, Astraline, Auralite 23, Azeztulite, Blue Flint, Brandenberg Amethyst, Celestite, Celestobarite, Chevron Amethyst, Citrine, Danburite, Dianite, Diaspore (Zultanite), Elestial Quartz, Fire and Ice, Fire and Ice and Nirvana Quartz, Golden Enhydro Herkimer, Golden Himalayan Azeztulite, Green Ridge Quartz, Hematite, Herkimer Diamond, Holly Agate, Keyiapo, Khutnohorite, Kunzite, Lapis Lazuli, Lavender Quartz, Merkabite Calcite, Muscovite, Natrolite, Novaculite, Nuummite, Onyx, Orange River Quartz, Petalite, Phenacite, Phenacite in Feldspar, Prophecy Stone, Purple Siberian Quartz, Purpurite, Quartz, Rainbow Mayanite, Rosophia, Satyamani and Satyaloka Quartz, Scolecite, Selenite, Shungite, Snowflake Obsidian, Spirit Quartz, Stellar Beam Calcite, Sugilite, Tangerine Aura Quartz, Tanzanite, Tanzine Aura Quartz, Titanite (Sphene), Trigonic Quartz, Vera Cruz Amethyst, Violane, White Elestial. *Chakra:* soul star, foot or so above head

balance and align: Anandalite, Vera Cruz Amethyst, Violane

spin too rapid/stuck open: Celestobarite, Novaculite, Nuummite, Pinky-beige Ussingite, White, Rose or Smoky Elestial Quartz

spin too sluggish/stuck closed: Golden Himalayan Azeztulite, Petalite, Phenacite, Rosophia

---

Unless otherwise directed, apply crystal over chakras, organ or site of symptom, wear as jewellery, bathe with or use as crystal essence.

Spleen chakra: Amber, Aventurine, Bloodstone, Carnelian, Chlorite Quartz, Emerald, Eye of the Storm, Fire Opal, Flint, Gaspeite, Green Fluorite, Jade, Orange River Quartz, Prasiolite, Rhodochrosite, Rhodonite, Ruby, Tugtupite, Zircon. *Chakra:* under left armpit

> **balance and align:** Charoite, Emerald, Eye of the Storm, Flint, Green Aventurine, Tugtupite
>
> **clear attachments and hooks:** Aventurine, Chert, Flint, Gaspeite, Jade, Jasper, Lemurian Seed
>
> **for the right armpit:** Bloodstone, Eye of the Storm, Gaspeite, Triplite, Tugtupite
>
> **spin too rapid/stuck open:** Amber, Aventurine, Chlorite Quartz, Eye of the Storm, Flint, Gaspeite, Green Fluorite, Jade, Prasiolite, Tugtupite
>
> **spin too sluggish/stuck closed:** Fire Opal, Orange River Quartz, Rhodonite, Ruby, Topaz

Stellar Gateway chakra: Afghanite, Ajoite, Amethyst Elestial, Amphibole, Anandalite™, Angelinite, Angel's Wing Calcite, Apophyllite, Astraline, Azeztulite, Brandenberg Amethyst, Celestite, Dianite, Diaspore (Zultanite), Elestial Quartz, Fire and Ice, Golden Himalayan Azeztulite, Golden Selenite, Green Ridge Quartz, Holly Agate, Ice Quartz, Kunzite, Merkabite Calcite, Moldavite, Nirvana Quartz, Novaculite, Petalite, Phenacite, Purpurite, Stellar Beam Calcite, Titanite (Sphene), Trigonic Quartz, White Elestial Quartz. *Chakra:* arm's length above head.

Unless otherwise directed, apply crystal over chakras, organ or site of symptom, wear as jewellery, bathe with or use as crystal essence.

balance and align: Ajoite, Anandalite, Amethyst Elestial, Brandenberg Amethyst, Kunzite

spin too rapid/stuck open: Amphibole Quartz, Ice Quartz, Merkabite Calcite, Pinky-beige Ussingite, Purpurite

spin too sluggish/stuck closed: Angel's Wing Calcite, Diaspore, Phenacite

Third Eye (brow) chakra: Afghanite, Ajoite, Ajo Quartz, Amber, Amechlorite, Amethyst, Ammolite, Amphibole Quartz, Angelite, Apophyllite, Aquamarine, Axinite, Azurite, Black Moonstone, Blue Calcite, Blue Kyanite, Blue Lace Agate, Blue Obsidian, Blue Selenite, Blue Topaz, Blue Tourmaline, Bytownite (Yellow Labradorite), Cacoxenite, Cavansite, Champagne Aura Quartz, Diaspore, Electric-blue Obsidian, Eye of the Storm, Garnet, Glaucophane, Golden Himalayan Azeztulite, Herderite, Herkimer Diamond, Holly Agate, Howlite, Indigo Aurum, Iolite, Kunzite, Labradorite, Lapis Lazuli, Lavender-purple Opal, Lazulite, Lepidolite, Libyan Gold Tektite, Malachite with Azurite (use as polished stone, make essence by indirect method), Moldavite, Pietersite, Purple Fluorite, Rhomboid Selenite, Sapphire, Serpentine in Obsidian, Sodalite, Spectrolite, Stilbite, Sugilite, Tangerine Aura Quartz, Turquoise, Unakite, Yellow Labradorite (Bytownite). *Chakra:* above and between eyebrows

   balance and align: Anandalite, Sugilite

spin too rapid/stuck open: Diaspore, Iolite, Lavender-purple Opal, Pietersite, Serpentine in Obsidian, Sodalite, Sugilite

spin too sluggish/stuck closed: Apophyllite, Azurite, Banded Agate, Diaspore, Herkimer Diamond, Optical Calcite, Rhomboid Calcite, Rhomboid Selenite, Royal Blue Sapphire, Tanzine Aura Quartz, Yellow Labradorite (Bytownite)

Throat chakra: Ajoite, Ajo Quartz, Amber, Amethyst, Aquamarine, Astraline, Azurite, Blue Chalcedony, Blue Lace Agate, Blue Kyanite, Blue Obsidian, Blue Quartz, Blue Topaz, Blue Tourmaline, Chalcanthite, Chrysocolla, Chrysotile, Eye of the Storm, Glaucophane, Green Ridge Quartz, Indicolite Quartz, Kunzite, Lapis Lazuli, Lepidolite, Moldavite, Paraiba Tourmaline, Sugilite, Turquoise. Place over throat.

balance and align: Anandalite, Blue Chalcedony, Blue Lace Agate, Blue Topaz, Indicolite Quartz, Sapphire

spin too rapid/stuck open: Black Sapphire, Lepidolite, Paraiba Tourmaline, Sugilite, Turquoise

spin too sluggish/stuck closed: Chrysocolla, Lapis Lazuli, Moldavite, Turquoise

The Subtle Energy Bodies and Their Crystals

Ancestral: Anthrophyllite, Blue Holly Agate, Brandenberg Amethyst, Bumble Bee Jasper, Candle Quartz, Catlinite, Datolite, Eclipse Stone, Fairy Quartz, Icicle Calcite, Ilmenite, Jade, Kambaba Jasper, Lemurian Aquatine Calcite, Mohawkite, Peanut Wood, Petrified Wood, Porphyrite, Prasiolite, Rainbow Mayanite, Rainforest Jasper, Shaman Quartz, Smoky Elestial Quartz, Spirit Quartz, Starseed, Stromatolite. *Chakra:* soul star, past life, alta major, causal vortex, higher heart, earth star and Gaia gateway

Emotional: Apache Tear, Black Moonstone, Blue Moonstone, Botswana (Banded) Agate, Brandenberg Amethyst, Calcite, Danburite, Icicle Calcite, Kunzite, Lepidolite, Mangano Calcite, Moonstone, Pink Moonstone, Pink Petalite, Rainbow Mayanite, Rainbow Moonstone, Rainbow Obsidian, Rhodochrosite, Rhodonite, Rose Elestial Quartz, Rose Quartz, Rubellite, Selenite, Tourmalinated Quartz, Tugtupite, Watermelon

---

Unless otherwise directed, apply crystal over chakras, organ or site of symptom, wear as jewellery, bathe with or use as crystal essence.

Tourmaline. *Chakra:* solar plexus, three-chambered heart, sacral and base chakras, knees and feet

Etheric: Andescine Labradorite, Angelinite, Astraline, Brandenberg Amethyst, Chlorite Quartz, Chrysotile, Datolite, Elestial Quartz, Ethiopian Opal, Eye of the Storm, Flint, Girasol, Icicle Calcite, Keyiapo, Khutnohorite, Lemurian Aquitane Calcite, Poldervaarite, Pollucite, Quantum Quattro, Que Sera, Rainbow Mayanite, Rhodozite, Ruby Lavender Quartz, Sanda Rosa Azeztulite, Scheelite, Selenite, Shaman Quartz, Shungite, Stellar Beam Calcite, Tangerine Dream Lemurian, Tantalite. *Chakra:* seven traditional chakras, plus soma, past life, alta major, causal vortex

Karmic/karmic blueprint: Ammolite, Ammonite, Brandenberg Amethyst, Cloudy Quartz, Crinoidal Limestone, Datolite, Dumortierite, Flint, Kambaba Jasper, Keyiapo, Khutnohorite, Lemurian Seed, Nirvana Quartz, Rainbow Mayanite, Rhodozite, Ruby Lavender Quartz, Sanda Rosa Azeztulite, Scheelite, Shaman Quartz, Shungite, Stromatolite, Titanite (Sphene) and see page 276. *Chakra:* past life, alta major, Causal Vortex, soma, knee and earth star

Lightbody: Agnitite™, Anandalite™, Angel's Wing Calcite, Blue Moonstone, Brandenberg Amethyst, Chlorite Brandenberg, Eklogite, Erythrite, Golden

Coracalcite, Golden Healer Quartz, Golden Himalayan Azeztulite, Hackmanite, Himalayan Gold Azeztulite™, Lemurian Seed, Lilac-purple Coquimbite, Madagascan Red 'Celestial Quartz', Mahogany Sheen Obsidian, Merkabite Calcite, Natrolite, Nirvana Quartz, Opal Aura Quartz, Phantom Calcite, Phenacite, Pink Lemurian, Prophecy Stone, Rainbow Mayanite, Red Amethyst, Rutilated Quartz (Angel Hair), Rutile with Hematite, Satyaloka Quartz, Satyamani Quartz, Scolecite, Spirit Quartz, Sugar Blade Quartz, Tangerine Dream Lemurian, Tiffany Stone, Trigonic Quartz, Tugtupite, Vera Cruz Amethyst, Violet Ussingite. *Chakra:* soma, soul star, stellar gateway, Gaia gateway, alta major, causal vortex

Mental: Amechlorite, Amethyst, Arfvedsonite, Auralite 23, Brandenberg Amethyst, Celadonite, Chlorite Brandenberg, Crystal Cap Amethyst, Dumortierite, Fluorite, Lemurian Seed, Merkabite Calcite, Nuummite, Owyhee Blue Opal, Rainbow Covellite, Rainbow Mayanite, Sapphire, Scheelite, Scolecite, Sodalite, Sugilite, Vera Cruz Amethyst. *Chakra:* third eye, soma, alta major, causal vortex

Physical, subtle: Amechlorite, Anandalite, Bloodstone, Brandenberg Amethyst, Carnelian, Cradle of Life Stone, Dumortierite, Eklogite, Eilat Stone, Flint, Hematite, Kambaba Jasper, Madagascan Red 'Celestial Quartz',

Unless otherwise directed, apply crystal over chakras, organ or site of symptom, wear as jewellery, bathe with or use as crystal essence.

Quantum Quattro, Que Sera, Rainbow Mayanite, Red Amethyst, Stromatolite. *Chakra:* base, sacral, dantien, earth star

Planetary: Aswan Granite, Brandenberg Amethyst, Charoite, Lapis Lazuli, Libyan Gold Tektite, Moldavite, Nebula Stone, Preseli Bluestone, Rainbow Mayanite, Starseed Quartz, Tektite. *Chakra:* past life, alta major, causal vortex, soma, stellar and Gaia gateway chakras

Spiritual: Anandalite, Azeztulite, Brandenberg Amethyst, Golden Herkimer Diamond, Golden Quartz, Green Ridge Quartz, Larimar, Lemurian Seed, Nirvana Quartz, Phenacite, Rainbow Mayanite, Shaman Quartz, Trigonic Amethyst, Trigonic Quartz. *Chakra:* past life, soul star, stellar gateway, alta major, causal vortex

Kundalini, Organs, Conditions and Healing Crystals

– A –

Acceptance of physical body: Celestobarite, Empowerite, Keyiapo, Llanite (Llanoite), Riebekite with Sugilite and Bustamite, Schalenblende, Thompsonite and see Incarnation page 270. *Chakra:* earth star, base, dantien, crown

Activate all chakras: Anandalite™, Brookite, Fulgarite, Golden Healer Quartz, Green Ridge Quartz, Phlogopite, Rhodozite, Triplite, Victorite and see Chakras page 233 and individual chakra entries

Adrenals: Aventurine, Axinite, Epidote, Eye of the Storm, Gaspeite, Jade, Nunderite, Picrolite, Richterite. *Chakra:* base, dantien, solar plexus

    balancing: Fire Opal, Rose Quartz, Yellow Labradorite

    calming: Cacoxenite, Eye of the Storm, Fire Opal, Green Calcite, Jamesonite, Kyanite, Richterite, Rose Quartz, Yellow Labradorite

Unless otherwise directed, apply crystal over chakras, organ or site of symptom, wear as jewellery, bathe with or use as crystal essence.

overload: Axinite, Eye of the Storm, Jade, Richterite

Aggression, calm: Rose Quartz, Serpentine with Seraphinite

Akashic Record, read: Blue Aventurine, Brandenberg Amethyst, Cathedral Quartz, Celestobarite, Chrysotile, Optical Calcite, Prehnite, Stichtite, Tanzanite, Tibetan Black Spot Quartz, Trigonic Quartz. *Chakra:* past life, third eye, crown and see Past life healing page 301

Align:

> **all chakras, especially third eye and crown or higher crown to the lightbody through the soul star:** Vera Cruz Amethyst
>
> **balance and activate base through to heart chakras:** Bloodstone, Carnelian, Green Ridge Quartz, Triplite
>
> **lightbody to the physical body through the lower chakra system and to the divine through the higher vibration chakras:** Golden Coracalcite
>
> **mind-body-spirit:** Aurichalcite, Eye of the Storm, Golden Coracalcite, Green Ridge Quartz, Larvikite, Sillimanite. *Chakra:* alta major (base of skull) and dantien
>
> **physical and subtle bodies:** Alexandrite, Anandalite™, Aurichalcite, Empowerite, Fulgarite, Golden Coracalcite, Golden Healer, Green Ridge Quartz, Herderite, Lemurian Seed, Mount Shasta Opal, Nuummite, Paraiba Tourmaline, Schalenblende, Scheelite, Sillimanite, Thompsonite, Zincite. *Chakra:* alta major (base of skull), soma

Unless otherwise directed, apply crystal over chakras, organ or site of symptom, wear as jewellery, bathe with or use as crystal essence.

the chakras: Afghanite, Amber, Anandalite™, Annabergite, Barite, Black Kyanite, Chrysoprase, Citrine, Gaia Stone, Kyanite, Lemurian Seed, Lepidicrosite, Paraiba Tourmaline, Picrolite, Pink Kunzite, Quartz, Shungite, Sichuan Quartz, Sillimanite, Sodalite, and see pages 194–208. *Chakra:* earth star to higher crown, dantien

> **physical with multidimensional consciousness:** Citrine
>
> **with etheric bodies:** Anandalite
>
> **with lightbody:** Anandalite, Green Ridge Quartz
>
> **with physical body:** Amber, Anandalite, Shungite

Ancestral:

> **DNA:** Brandenberg Amethyst, Datolite, Eye of the Storm, Icicle Calcite, Petrified Wood, Pyrite in Quartz, Snakeskin Pyrite, Stromatolite. *Chakra:* past life, alta major (base of skull)
>
> **issues:** Porphyrite (Chinese Letter Stone). *Chakra:* past life or alta major
>
> **line, healing:** Brandenberg Amethyst, Candle Quartz, Chlorite Quartz, Crinoidal Limestone, Datolite, Fairy Quartz, Ilmenite, Lemurian Aquitane Calcite, Mohawkite, Prasiolite, Rainforest Jasper, Shaman Quartz, Smoky Elestial Quartz, Spirit Quartz. *Chakra:* past life, base
>
> **patterns:** Anthrophyllite, Arfvedsonite, Candle Quartz, Celadonite, Crinoidal Limestone, Eclipse Stone, Garnet in Quartz, Glendonite, Green Ridge

Quartz, Holly Agate, Mohawkite, Porphyrite (Chinese Letter Stone), Prasiolite, Rainbow Covellite, Rainbow Mayanite, Shaman Quartz with Chlorite, Scheelite, Starseed Quartz. *Chakra:* past life or alta major

Anchor:

both sections: Black/brown Flint, Black Kyanite, Blue Flint, Blue Moonstone, Brandenberg Amethyst, Celestobarite, Fulgarite, Gaia Stone, Goethite, Lemurian Jade, Hackmanite, Huebnerite, Kakortokite, Nebula Stone, Nuummite, Prasiolite, Preseli Bluestone, Rutile/Rutilated Quartz, Shaman Quartz, Specular Hematite, Smoky Rose Quartz, White Flint. *Chakra:* base, earth star, Gaia gateway, soma, crown, stellar gateway

cosmic: Azeztulite, Blue Moonstone, Brandenberg Amethyst, Faden Quartz, Flint, Hematite, Kakortokite, Lemurian Jade, Lemurian Seed, Menalite, Prasiolite, Preseli Bluestone, Rutile, Rutilated Quartz, Smoky Elestial Quartz, Smoky Rose Quartz, Specular Hematite, Starseed Quartz, Stellar Beam Calcite, Stibnite, Trigonic Quartz. *Chakra:* soma, crown, stellar gateway

shamanic (Earth): Black Tourmaline, Boji Stones, Calcite Fairy Stone, Celestobarite, Flint, Fulgarite, Gaia Stone, Hematite, Kakortokite, Lemurian Jade, Leopardskin Jasper, Menalite, Obsidian, Rainforest Jasper, Serpentine, Smoky Brandenberg, Smoky Elestial Quartz, Smoky Quartz. *Chakra:* dantien, sacral, base, earth star, Gaia gateway

Anchor expanded awareness: Brandenberg, Flint, Rhodozite, Trigonic Quartz with Tugtupite or Z-stone and see grounding stones page 261. *Chakra:* earth star, Gaia gateway

Anger, ameliorate: Cinnabar in Jasper, Ethiopian Opal, Nzuri Moyo. *Chakra:* base, dantien

Antisocial behaviour/aggression: Amethyst, Blizzard Stone, Bloodstone, Carnelian, Eye of the Storm, Rose Quartz, Ruby, Sardonyx, Selenite, Sodalite. Place in environment or around bed.

Antispasmodic: Aragonite, Azurite, Chrome Diopside, Diopside, Magnesite

Anxiety: Amber, Aventurine, Chrysoprase, Emerald, Galaxyite, Green Calcite, Hematite, Lemurian Aquitane Calcite, Lemurian Gold Opal, Khutnohorite, Kunzite, Labradorite, Moonstone, Nzuri Moyo, Oceanite, Owyhee Blue Opal, Pyrite, Pyrite in Magnesite, Riebekite with Sugilite and Bustamite, Rose Quartz, Rutilated Quartz, Scolecite, Smithsonite, Strawberry Quartz, Tanzanite, Thunder Egg, Tiger's Eye, Tourmaline, Tremolite, Tugtupite. *Chakra:* earth star, base

Arrogance: Covellite, Diopside. *Chakra:* base and soma

Astral projection/journeying: Afghanite, Apophyllite, Nuummite, Scolecite, Sedona Stone, Stibnite, Titanite (Sphene). Chakra: third eye, soma, crown, and see Journeying page 275 and travel page 291

    facilitate: double-terminated crystals, Preseli

Bluestone. *Chakra:* hold or apply to soma/third eye

prevention: Banded Agate, Faden Quartz (wear constantly at night or place by bed)

protection during: Nunderite, Stibnite (hold or wear)

Aura: Anandalite™, Beryllonite, Charoite, Flint, Quartz, Scolecite. Hold in front of solar plexus or sweep aura.

align with physical body: Ajo Blue Calcite, Amber, Anandalite, Candle Quartz, Empowerite, Fulgarite, Larvikite, Schalenblende, Scheelite, Scolecite, Sichuan Quartz, Sillimanite, Thompsonite. Hold over head or solar plexus.

blockages, remove: Ajo Quartz, Anandalite, Arfvedsonite, Beryllonite, Charoite, Fire and Ice Quartz, Flint, Fulgarite, Jasper, Prehnite with Epidote, Rainbow Mayanite, Rhodozite, Serpentine in Obsidian

cleansing: Amber, Amechlorite, Anandalite, Black Kyanite, Bloodstone, Citrine Spirit Quartz, Fire and Ice Quartz, Flint, Fulgarite, Green Jasper, Herkimer Diamond, Holly Agate, Keyiapo, Lepidocrosite, Mystic Topaz, Nuummite, Phlogopite, Pumice, Pyrite and Sphalerite, Pyrite in Quartz, Quartz, Rainbow Mayanite, Rutile, Smoky Quartz. 'Comb' aura thoroughly.

energize: Andandalite™, Gold in Quartz, Iolite, Quartz, Rainbow Mayanite, Sichuan Quartz, Triplite. *Chakra:* solar plexus

energy leakage, guard against: Eudialyte, Gaspeite,

Healer's Gold, Labradorite, Pyrite in Quartz, Quartz with Mica, Spectrolite. *Chakra:* higher heart. Wear constantly.

heal: Anandalite, Keyiapo, Piemontite, Scolecite, Sichuan Quartz, Smoky Amethyst, Tugtupite

'holes'/breaks: Aegirine, Amethyst, Aqua Aura, Brookite, Chinese Red Quartz, Eye of the Storm, Flint, Green Ridge Quartz, Green Tourmaline, Labradorite, Lemurian Seed, Quartz, Scolecite, Selenite. Place over site.

negativity, remove: Amber, Apache Tear, Black Jade, Fulgarite, Nuummite with Novaculite, Smoky Amethyst, Spectrolite, Tantalite. *Chakra:* solar plexus

protect: Amber, Amethyst, Apache Tear, Brandenberg Amethyst, Diamond, Honey Phantom Calcite, Hackmanite, Labradorite, Mahogany Sheen Obsidian, Master Shamanite, Nunderite, Orgonite, Paraiba Tourmaline, Quartz, Shattuckite with Ajoite, Tantalite. *Chakra:* higher heart. Wear continuously.

seal: Actinolite, Andean Blue Opal, Brookite, Feather Pyrite, Fulgarite, Galaxyite, Healer's Gold, Honey Phantom Calcite, Labradorite, Lorenzenite (Ramsayite), Molybdenite in Quartz, Nunderite, Pyromorphite, Serpentine in Obsidian, Smoky Amethyst, Spectrolite, Tantalite, Thunder Egg, Valentinite and Stibnite, Xenotine

stabilize: Agate, Fulgarite, Granite, Labradorite, Mtrolite, Poppy Jasper. *Chakra:* earth star

strengthen: Ajo Blue Calcite, Anandalite, Brookite,

Unless otherwise directed, apply crystal over chakras, organ or site of symptom, wear as jewellery, bathe with or use as crystal essence.

Ethiopian Opal, Flint, Magnetite (Lodestone), Quartz Tantalite, Thunder Egg, Zircon

weakness, overcome: Brookite, Zircon

Autism/hyperactivity: Cerussite, Charoite, Moldavite, Sugilite. *Chakra:* earth, base, solar plexus. Wear continuously or keep in pocket.

Autoimmune diseases: Bastnasite, Bloodstone, Brandenberg Amethyst, Chinese Red Quartz, Diaspore (Zultanite), Gabbro, Granite, Mookaite Jasper, Paraiba Tourmaline, Quantum Quattro, Que Sera, Richterite, Rosophia, Shungite, Tangerose, Titanite (Sphene), Winchite. *Chakra:* dantien, higher heart

Autonomic nervous system: Alexandrite, Amazonite, Amber, Ametrine, Anglesite, Aventurine, Bloodstone, Charoite, Merlinite, Quantum Quattro, Que Sera, Sunstone, Tourmaline. *Chakra:* dantien

– B –

Back:

> **ache:** Amber, Bloodstone, Blue Agate, Cathedral Quartz, Hematite, Iolite, Magnetite, Que Sera, Sapphire
>
> **disc elasticity:** Aragonite
>
> **pain:** Cathedral Quartz (over site of pain), Lapis Lazuli, Magnetite (Lodestone), Que Sera, Rutilated Quartz, Sapphire. *Chakra:* base, sacral, solar plexus or over site

Baggage, releasing emotional: Chrysotile in Serpentine, Cumberlandite, Eclipse Stone, Garnet in Quartz, Graphic Smoky Quartz (Zebra Stone), Mount Shasta Opal, Tangerose, Tanzine Aura Quartz, Tremolite, Tugtupite, Wind Fossil Agate, Xenotine. *Chakra:* solar plexus, heart, causal vortex

Balance:

> **all chakras:** Anandalite, Citrine, Pink Kunzite, Sunstone and see Chakras page 233
>
> **body-mind-spirit:** Actinolite, Larvikite, Merlinite
>
> **male/female energies:** Alexandrite, Amphibole Quartz, Day and Night Quartz, Khutnohorite. *Chakra:* base and sacral
>
> **physical body with etheric:** Ajoite, Andara Glass, Astraline, Eye of the Storm, Granite, Larvikite, Nuummite, Rutile with Hematite, Sanda Rosa Azeztulite, Mohawkite, Thompsonite

Unless otherwise directed, apply crystal over chakras, organ or site of symptom, wear as jewellery, bathe with or use as crystal essence.

physical body with lightbody: Golden Coracalcite, Golden Healer Quartz, Prophecy Stone, Red Celestial Madagascan Quartz, Scheelite, Scolecite, Victorite

vibrational shifts: Anandalite™, Lemurian Gold Opal, Lemurian Seed

yin-yang: Amphibole, Dalmatian Stone, Day and Night Quartz, Eilat Stone, Merlinite, Morion, Poppy Jasper, Shiva Lingam, Spirit Quartz. *Chakra:* sacral, dantien (or wear continuously)

Biomagnetic field destabilized: Ajoite, Anandalite, Flint, Galena (wash hands after use, make essence by indirect method), Hematite, Kyanite, Lepidolite, Magnetite, Orgonite, Preseli Bluestone, Quartz, Shungite, Sodalite. *Chakra:* dantien, solar plexus, and see Aura page 218

realign/strengthen: Angelinite, Astraline, Ethiopian Opal, Flint, Galena (wash hands after use, make essence by indirect method), Golden Healer Quartz, Gold in Quartz, Magnetite, Poldervaarite, Pollucite, Preseli Bluestone, Quantum Quattro, Que Sera, Shungite, Sodalite

Bipolar disorder/extreme mood swings: Bastnasite, Brucite, Charoite, Halite, Kunzite, Larimar, Lepidocrosite, Montebrasite, Peridot, Tantalite. *Chakra:* third eye

Bladder: Amber, Bloodstone, Jade, Jasper, Orange Calcite, Prehnite, Topaz, Tourmaline, Vanadinite (make essence by indirect method), Yellow Sapphire

---

Unless otherwise directed, apply crystal over chakras, organ or site of symptom, wear as jewellery, bathe with or use as crystal essence.

Blockages:

> **clear:** Anandalite, Azurite, Black Opal Bloodstone, Clear Quartz, Flint, Lapis Lazuli
>
> **self-imposed, remove:** Bowenite (New Jade), Brandenberg, Elestial Quartz, Gold Siberian Quartz, Prehnite with Epidote, Rhodozite, Serpentine in Obsidian, Sichuan Quartz. *Chakra:* higher heart

Blocked feelings: Indicolite Quartz, Lepidocrosite, Malachite, Mangano Calcite, Montebrasite, Obsidian, Peridot, Pyrite and Sphalerite, Pyrite in Quartz, Rainbow Mayanite, Tantalite, Tanzine Aura Quartz. *Chakra:* third eye

Blood: Bloodstone, Cinnabar, Garnet, Sonora Sunrise, red stones. *Chakra:* heart, spleen

> **cells, red to white ratio:** Fuchsite, Tiger Iron
>
> **circulation:** Amethyst, Bloodstone, Carnelian, Galena (wash hands after use, make essence by indirect method), Garnet, Pink Tourmaline, Ruby, Seraphinite, Sodalite
>
> **cleanser:** Amethyst, Ametrine, Aquamarine, Bloodstone, Chlorite Quartz, Garnet, Hematite, Lapis Lazuli, Mookaite, Ruby, Tourmaline. *Chakra:* spleen
>
> **clots, dissolve:** Amethyst, Bloodstone, Hematite
>
> **clotting, improve:** Calcite, Red Chalcedony, Sapphire, Shattuckite
>
> **disorders:** Amethyst, Bloodstone, Blue Quartz, Cherry Opal, Chrysocolla, Fulgarite, Lapis Lazuli, Magnetite (Lodestone), Mookaite, Onyx, Prehnite,

Sapphire

excessive clotting: Magnesite

faulty oxygenation: Amethyst, Carnelian, Chrysocolla, Kambaba Jasper, Stromatolite

flow in liver: Albite, Gaspeite, Mookaite, Variscite

poisoning: Carnelian, Quantum Quattro

purification: Angelite, Bloodstone, Pink Tourmaline, Sapphire

vessels: Fluorite, Fulgarite, Merlinite, Topaz

Blood pressure:

equalize: Aventurine, Charoite, Tourmaline. *Chakra:* heart, solar plexus

high: Amethyst, Bloodstone, Blue Chalcedony, Charoite, Chrysocolla, Chrysoprase, Dioptase, Emerald, Jade, Kyanite, Labradorite, Lapis Lazuli, Malachite (use as polished stone, make essence by indirect method), Rhodochrosite, Sodalite. *Chakra:* heart

low: Carnelian, Red Calcite, Rhodochrosite, Ruby, Sodalite, Tourmaline. *Chakra:* heart

Blood sugar imbalances: Astraline, Chinese Chromium Quartz, Chrome Diopside, Citrine, Green Shaman Quartz, Huebnerite, Malacholla, Maw Sit Sit, Mtrolite, Muscovite, Orange Kyanite, Owyhee Blue Opal, Peridot, Pink Opal, Pink Sunstone, Rose Quartz, Serpentine in Obsidian, Shungite, Sodalite, Stichtite and Serpentine, Tugtupite and see Diabetes page 246 and Pancreas page 300. *Chakra:* spleen, dantien, heart

---

Unless otherwise directed, apply crystal over chakras, organ or site of symptom, wear as jewellery, bathe with or use as crystal essence.

Blown chakra: Fire Agate, Lemurian Seed

Blueprint, etheric: Anandalite, Andescine Labradorite, Astraline, Beryllonite, Black Kyanite, Brandenberg Amethyst, Chlorite Quartz, Ethiopian Opal, Eye of the Storm, Fulgarite, Keyiapo, Khutnohorite, Lemurian Aquitane Calcite, Pollucite, Rhodozite, Ruby Lavender Quartz, Sanda Rosa Azeztulite, Scheelite, Seriphos Quartz, Tantalite. *Chakra:* soma

Body:

  acceptance of: Candle Quartz, Eye of the Storm, Phenacite, Vanadinite (make essence by indirect method). *Chakra:* earth, base, crown

  discomfort at being in: Candle Quartz, Pearl Spar Dolomite, Quantum Quattro, Strontianite. *Chakra:* earth star, base, sacral, dantien

  fluids, balance: Azeztulite with Morganite, Bastnasite, Hackmanite, Nunderite, Scheelite, Smoky Amethyst, Trigonic Quartz. *Chakra:* earth star, base, sacral

  heat, excess: Brazilianite. *Chakra:* earth star, base, sacral

  promote repair: Bixbite, Rutilated Quartz, Seraphinite, Tantalite, and see cellular healing page 231. *Chakra:* earth star, base, sacral

  rebalance: Shungite with Steatite, Victorite

  strengthen: Blue Aragonite, Candle Quartz, Erythrite, Fiskenaesset Ruby, Peridot, Poppy Jasper. *Chakra:* earth star, base, sacral, dantien

Unless otherwise directed, apply crystal over chakras, organ or site of symptom, wear as jewellery, bathe with or use as crystal essence.

work efficiently: Golden Healer Quartz, Phlogopite

Bones: Brookite, Cat's Eye Quartz, Cradle of Life, Cryolite, Feather Pyrite, Fluorapatite, Golden Coracalcite, Hausmanite, Khutnohorite, Marialite, Petrified Wood, Piemontite, Poldervaarite, Pyrite in Magnesite, Scolecite, Shell Jasper, Stone of Dreams, Strontianite, Titanite (Sphene), Wind Fossil Agate

> **aching:** Cradle of Life
>
> **brittle:** Faden Quartz, Fire and Ice Quartz, Pink Crackle Quartz, Scolecite, Trummer Jasper
>
> **broken:** Axinite, Creedite, Faden Quartz, Glendonite, Graphic Smoky Quartz (Zebra Stone), Nzuri Moyo, Oligocrase
>
> **disease:** Zebra Stone
>
> **disorders:** Graphic Smoky Quartz, Scolecite
>
> **growth:** Cavansite, Diaspore (Zultanite), Khutnohorite, Piemontite
>
> **healing:** Cradle of Life, Eilat Stone
>
> **loss:** Cavansite
>
> **marrow:** Erythrite, Goethite
>
> **strengthening:** Glendonite, Graphic Smoky Quartz, Pink Crackle Quartz, Scolecite
>
> **structure:** Cradle of Life, Graphic Smoky Quartz, Hausmanite, Khutnohorite

Boundaries: Brazilianite, Lemurian Jade, Serpentine in Obsidian, Tantalite. *Chakra:* solar plexus (or wear continuously)

Bowels: Xenotine. *Chakra:* dantien

Unless otherwise directed, apply crystal over chakras, organ or site of symptom, wear as jewellery, bathe with or use as crystal essence.

blockage: Ajoite with Shattukite, Pyrite and Sphalerite, Pyrite in Quartz, Rhodozite, Rosophia

Brain: Amber, Amethyst, Beryl, Botswana Agate, Brandenberg Amethyst, Carnelian, Crystal Cap Amethyst, Epidote, Green Tourmaline, Kyanite, Labradorite, Magnesite, Nuummite, Prehnite with Epidote, Pyrite and Sphalerite, Royal Sapphire, Schalenblende, Sodalite, Staurolite, Trigonic Quartz, White Heulandite, Vera Cruz Amethyst. *Chakra:* third eye, soma, crown, alta major

> **balance left-right hemispheres:** Crystal Cap Amethyst, Cumberlandite, Eudialyte, Hematite with Rutile, Lilac Quartz, Rhodozite, Sodalite, Stromatolite, Sugilite, Trigonic Quartz. *Chakra:* soma
>
> **blood flow, improve:** Iron Pyrite
>
> **chemistry:** Barite, Stichtite
>
> **damage:** Amphibole, Anthrophyllite, Brandenberg Amethyst, Galaxyite, Herderite
>
> **degeneration:** Anthrophyllite, Sodalite
>
> **detox:** Amechlorite, Chlorite Quartz, Eye of the Storm, Klinoptilolith, Lapis Lazuli, Larvikite, Nuummite, Rainbow Covellite, Rhodozite, Richterite, Ruby, Shungite, Smoky Quartz with Aegirine, Sodalite, Thulite, Zircon
>
> **disorders:** Brandenberg Amethyst, Chalcopyrite, Galaxyite, Holly Agate, Khutnohorite, Sapphire, Sodalite, Stilbite
>
> **dysfunction:** Anthrophyllite, Blue Holly Agate,

Cryolite, Cumberlandite, Sodalite

fatigue: Apricot Quartz, Pyrite in Quartz, Strawberry Lemurian, Turquoise

function: Cryolite, Phantom Calcite, Rhodozite

neural pathways: Anglesite, Celestobarite, Crystal Cap Amethyst, Feather Calcite, Feather Pyrite, Holly Agate, Larvikite, Phantom Calcite, Pyrite and Sphalerite, Schalenblende, Scolecite, Stichtite

stem: Blue Moonstone, Chrysotile, Chrysotile in Serpentine, Cradle of Life, Eye of the Storm, Kambaba Jasper, Schalenblende, Stromatolite

synapses: Azurite, Moss Agate

Breathing disorders: Blue Aragonite, Blue Crackle Quartz, Hanksite, Morganite, Moss Agate, Riebekite with Sugilite and Bustamite, Tremolite, Vanadinite (make essence by indirect method). *Chakra:* dantien, heart

Breathlessness: Amber, Amethyst, Apophyllite, Black Onyx, Jet, Kambaba Jasper, Magnetite (Lodestone), Morganite, Moss Agate, Quantum Quattro, Que Sera, Stromatolite, Vanadinite (make essence by indirect method). *Chakra:* higher heart, solar plexus, throat

Burning sensation: Lilac Quartz, Rose Quartz

Burn-out: Carnelian, Crackled Fire Agate, Marcasite, Poppy Jasper, Quantum Quattro, Que Sera, Red Jasper, Strawberry Lemurian. *Chakra:* base, dantien

– C –

Calming:

    emotions: Mount Shasta Opal, Oceanite, Tugtupite

    fear: Arsenopyrite, Eilat Stone, Graphic Smoky Quartz (Zebra Stone), Guardian Stone, Khutnohorite, Oceanite, Scolecite, Tangerose, Thunder Egg

    physical body: Jamesonite, Scolecite. *Chakra:* dantien

Capillaries: Feather Pyrite, Moss Agate

Cardiovascular system: Kunzite, Peridot and see Heart page 264

Causes of dis-ease:

    anxiety or fear: Candle Quartz, Dumortierite, Eilat Stone, Khutnohorite, Oceanite, Tangerose, Thunder Egg, Tremolite, Tugtupite. *Chakra:* solar plexus

    damaged immune system: Blizzard Stone, Brandenberg Amethyst, Diaspore (Zultanite), Gabbro, Lemurian Jade, Mookaite Jasper, Nzuri Moyo, Ocean Blue Jasper, Pyrite and Sphalerite, Quantum Quattro, Que Sera, Schalenblende, Shungite, Stone of Solidarity, Super 7, Tangerose, Titanite (Sphene), Winchite. *Chakra:* dantien, higher heart

    emotional exhaustion: Candle Quartz, Mount Shasta Opal, Prehnite with Epidote. *Chakra:* solar plexus

    mental stress: Candle Quartz, Eye of the Storm, Guinea Fowl Jasper, Lemurian Gold Opal, Richterite, Shungite. *Chakra:* third eye, soma

    negative attitudes or emotions: Candle Quartz,

Unless otherwise directed, apply crystal over chakras, organ or site of symptom, wear as jewellery, bathe with or use as crystal essence.

Kornerupine, Pyrite in Quartz, Thunder Egg

past life: Dumortierite and see Past life healing page 301

shock, trauma or psychic attack: Apricot Quartz, Empowerite, Guardian Stone, Linerite, Mohave Turquoise, Mohawkite, Oceanite, Polychrome Jasper, Richterite, Ruby Lavender Quartz, Tantalite, Victorite

stress and tension: Basalt, Bird's Eye Jasper, Bustamite, Eye of the Storm, Marble, Richterite, Riebekite with Sugilite and Bustamite, Shungite, Tugtupite

underlying, discover: Faden Quartz, Indicolite Quartz, Pholocomite

Cells: Celestite, Dioptase, Garnet, Herkimer Diamond, Iron Pyrite, Staurolite, Yellow Kunzite

detox: Chlorite Quartz, Eye of the Storm, Fulgarite, Klinoptilolith, Larvikite, Seraphinite, Shungite, Smoky Quartz with Aegirine

energetic balance: Lemurian Gold Opal, Rainbow Covellite, Richterite, Sanda Rosa Azeztulite, Shungite. *Chakra:* dantien

metabolism: Ammolite, Pyrite in Magnesite, Sardonyx, Tangerine Sun Aura Quartz

production: Bixbite, Tantalite. *Chakra:* higher heart

rejuvenation: Jasper, Rhodonite, Sodalite

repair: Bixbite, Glendonite, Rosophia, Rutilated Quartz

walls: Calcite Fairy Stone, Eye of the Storm, Feather

Pyrite, Poppy Jasper, Titanite (Sphene). *Chakra:* dantien

Cellular:

blueprint: Ajoite, Ajo Quartz, Brandenberg Amethyst, Chlorite Quartz, Eye of the Storm, Fulgarite, Keyiapo, Khutnohorite, Rainbow Mayanite, Rhodozite, Ruby Lavender Quartz, Scheelite, Seriphos Quartz, Shattuckite, Yellow Kunzite. *Chakra:* higher heart, soma, alta major (base of skull) and see Karmic and Etheric bodies page 210

detoxification: Chlorite Quartz, Eye of the Storm, Fulgarite, Kambaba Jasper, Larvikite, Rainbow Covellite, Richterite, Seraphinite, Shieldite, Shungite, Smoky Quartz with Aegirine, Stromatolite, Tantalite

disorders: Biotite, Celestite, Dioptase, Eye of the Storm, Garnet, Herkimer Diamond, Iron Pyrite, Pollucite, Pyrite in Magnesite, Reinerite, Rhodozite, Seraphinite, Shungite, Staurolite, Yellow Kunzite, Zoisite

disorganisation: Agnitite, Azotic Topaz, Biotite, Eklogite, Fulgarite, Golden Healer Quartz, Kambaba Jasper, Mangano Vesuvianite, Quantum Quattro, Que Sera, Reinerite, Rosophia, Sanda Rosa Azeztulite, Schalenblende, Shungite, Topaz

healing: Ajo Quartz, Brandenberg Amethyst, Crystal Cap Amethyst, Elestial Quartz, Eudialyte, Eye of the Storm, Khutnohorite, Mangano Vesuvianite, Marialite, Nebula Stone, Pyrite in Magnesite, Rainbow

Mayanite, Rainforest Jasper, Reinerite, Rhodozite, Rosophia, Schalenblende, Seraphinite, Tantalite, Titanite (Sphene), Zoisite

matrix: Eye of the Storm, Gold in Quartz

memory: Ajoite, Ajo Quartz, Andean Blue Opal, Azotic Topaz, Brandenberg Amethyst, Bustamite, Chrysotile, Datolite, Dumortierite, Eilat Stone, Elestial Quartz, Eye of the Storm, Heulandite, Lepidocrosite, Leopardskin Jasper, Nuummite, Rainbow Mayanite, Rhodozite, Sichuan Quartz, Smoky Quartz with Aegirine, Sodalite, Spirit Quartz, Valentinite and Stibnite. *Chakra:* dantien, alta major

micro level: Dendritic Agate, Fulgarite, Merlinite, Ruby Lavender Quartz, Seraphinite

processes: Eye of the Storm, Feather Pyrite

regeneration: Andean Blue Opal, Elestial Quartz, Eye of the Storm, Jasper, Lepidicrosite, Reinerite, Rhodonite, Rosophia, Seraphinite, Shungite, Sodalite, Tantalite, Zoisite

structure: Ajoite, Ajo Quartz, Bornite, Cradle of Life, Indicolite Tourmaline, Lilac Quartz, Hausmanite, Messina Quartz, Novaculite, Reinerite, Rhodozite, Selenite, Shattuckite, Shungite

wall reprogramming: Brandenberg Amethyst, Calcite Fairy Stone, Eye of the Storm, Feather Pyrite, Fulgarite, Poppy Jasper, Seraphinite, Shattuckite, Titanite (Sphene). *Chakra:* dantien

Central nervous system, depleted or disturbed:

Anandalite™, Alexandrite, Amethyst, Anglesite, Aventurine, Brandenberg Amethyst, Celestite, Dioptase, Fulgarite, Larvikite, Merlinite, Natrolite with Scolecite, Prehnite with Epidote, Rhodonite, Rose Quartz, Sodalite. *Chakra:* dantien. Wear continuously.

Centring: Bloodstone, Calcite, Celestobarite, Coral, Eye of the Storm, Flint, Fossilised Wood, Garnet, Hematite, Kunzite, Obsidian, Onyx, Peanut Wood, Quartz, Red Jasper, Ruby, Sardonyx, Tourmalinated Quartz

Cerebellum: Anthrophyllite, Kambaba Jasper, Kyanite, Shungite, Sodalite, Stromatolite. *Chakra:* third eye, crown

Cervix: Calcite Fairy Stone, Menalite. *Chakra:* sacral

Chakras:

See also individual chakra entries pages 194-208

    align: Anandalite, Auralite 23, Brochantite, Citrine, Fulgarite, Golden Healer Quartz, Green Ridge Quartz, Kyanite, Lemurian Seed, Montebrasite, Novaculite, Quartz, Rhodozite, Sillimanite

    align with physical body: Amber, Anandalite, Candle Quartz, Celestial Quartz, Fulgarite, Keyiapo, Lemurian Jade, Lemurian Seed, Morion, Prasiolite, Preseli Bluestone, Rainbow Mayanite, Rhodozite, Seraphinite, Sichuan Quartz, Sillimanite, Smoky Herkimer Diamond, Thompsonite

    balance: Anandalite, Auralite 23, Black Kyanite, Golden Healer Quartz, Lemurian Seed, Petalite, Seraphinite, Sichuan Quartz, Sunstone

    blockages: Ajo Quartz, Amechlorite, Anandalite

(Aurora Quartz), Azurite, Black Kyanite, Bloodstone, Charoite, Chlorite Quartz, Clear Quartz, Flint, Fulgarite, Golden Healer Quartz, Green Ridge Quartz, Jasper, Lapis Lazuli, Lemurian Seed, Picrolite, Prehnite with Epidote, Pyrite and Sphalerite, Quartz, Que Sera, Rainbow Mayanite, Rhodozite, Sanda Rosa Azeztulite

blown: Fire Agate

clean, protect and align all: Anandalite, Petrified Wood

cleanse: Amethyst, Anandalite, Black Kyanite, Bloodstone, Calcite, Celestite, Citrine, Enstatite and Diopside, Flint, Fulgarite, Garnet, Golden Healer Quartz, Graphic Smoky Quartz (Zebra Stone), Green Fluorite, Novaculite, Nuummite, Orange Kyanite, Pink Kunzite, Quartz, Rainbow Mayanite, Rhodozaz, Rhodozite, Scolecite, Sugilite, Tourmaline

connect higher: Angel's Wing Calcite, Astraline, Rhodozaz, Rosophia, Titanite (Sphene)

energy leakage, prevent: Ajoite with Shattuckite, Black Tourmaline, Eudialyte, Gaspeite, Green Aventurine, Healer's Gold, Hematite, Labradorite, Pyrite in Quartz, Quartz Tantalite, Thunder Egg. *Chakra:* dantien, spleen, solar plexus

entities, release from: Petalite, Smoky Amethyst

ground energies through: Aztee, Champagne Aura Quartz, Empowerite, Fulgarite, Keyiapo, Mohawkite, Peanut Wood, Polychrome Jasper, Red Amethyst,

Rhodozite, Schalenblende, Serpentine in Obsidian, Stromatolite, Thunder Egg. *Chakra:* earth star

holes, repair: Amethyst, Anandalite, Barite, Black Kyanite, Green Tourmaline, Lemurian Seed, Novaculite, Quartz, Rainbow Mayanite, Rutilated Quartz, Selenite

integrate higher: Anandalite, Fulgarite, Montebrasite, Petalite, Ruby Lavender Quartz™, Selenite, Titanite (Sphene)

mental influences, detach: Kunzite, Selenite

negative karma, disturbances from: Petalite

protect: Apache Tear, Eilat Stone, Jet, Labradorite, Mohawkite, Quartz, Richterite, Tantalite, Thunder Egg

remove blockages: Azurite, Bloodstone, Flint, Fulgarite, Green Ridge Quartz, Jasper, Lapis Lazuli, Lemurian Seed, Prehnite with Epidote, Pyrite and Sphalerite, Quartz, Rainbow Mayanite, Rhodozite, Selenite, Serpentine in Obsidian. *Chakra:* dantien

revitalize: Anandalite, Malacholla. *Chakra:* dantien

stimulate or sedate as necessary: Poppy Jasper. *Chakra:* dantien

strengthen: Magnetite (Lodestone), Quartz

Change:

assimilating: Actinolite, Basalt, Bismuth, Blue Euclase, Brandenberg Amethyst, Clevelandite, Conichalcite, Frondellite, Green Ridge Quartz, Luxullianite, Nunderite, Nuummite, Shift Crystal,

Tangerose. *Chakra:* heart, higher heart

facilitating: Ethiopian Opal, Eudialyte, Fluorapatite, Golden Danburite, Heulandite, Luxullianite, Merlinite, Phenacite in Red Feldspar, Quantum Quattro, Scapolite, Shaman Quartz, Snakeskin Pyrite, Tangerine Dream Lemurian. *Chakra:* heart

ground: Aztee, Basalt, Champagne Aura Quartz, Empowerite, Lemurian Jade, Libyan Gold Tektite, Mohawkite, Nunderite, Peanut Wood, Polychrome Jasper, Preseli Bluestone, Schalenblende, Serpentine in Obsidian. *Chakra:* earth star, dantien

metaphysical: Novaculite

of life: Menalite and see Menopause page 285.

psychological: Annabergite, Elestial Quartz, Lilac Crackle Quartz

riding out: Datolite, Flint, Gabbro, Huebnerite, Kakortokite, Luxullianite, Montebrasite, Mtrolite, Nunderite, Ocean Jasper, Preseli Bluestone

vibrational: Anandalite™, Bismuth, Candle Quartz, Ethiopian Opal, Lemurian Gold Opal, Sanda Rosa Azeztulite, Tangerose, Tugtupite with Nuummite

Chest: Hiddenite, Larimar, Prehnite. *Chakra:* heart

constriction: Chrysopal (Blue-green Opal), Quantum Quattro

pains: Amber, Dioptase, Emerald, Malachite (use as polished stone, make essence by indirect method), Rhodochrosite, Rhodonite, Rose Quartz, Rutilated Quartz

---

Unless otherwise directed, apply crystal over chakras, organ or site of symptom, wear as jewellery, bathe with or use as crystal essence.

Chills: Novaculite, Poppy Jasper, Pyrite in Magnesite

Chronic:

> **conditions:** Apricot Quartz, Bismuth, Diopside
>
> **dis-ease:** Apricot Quartz, Bismuth, Cathedral Quartz, Lemurian Jade, Orgonite, Petrified Wood, Quantum Quattro, Que Sera, Shungite, Witches Finger. *Chakra:* dantien
>
> **exhaustion:** Apricot Quartz, Bismuth, Bronzite, Cinnabar in Jasper, Eye of the Storm, Poppy Jasper, Prehnite with Epidote, Triplite, Trummer Jasper. *Chakra:* dantien, higher heart
>
> **fatigue syndrome:** Adamite, Amethyst, Ametrine, Apricot Quartz, Aquamarine, Aragonite, Barite, Chrysotile in Serpentine, Citrine, Green Tourmaline, Orange Calcite, Petrified Wood, Pyrite in Quartz, Quartz, Rhodochrosite, Ruby, Shungite, Tourmaline, Triplite, Trummer Jasper, Zincite. *Chakra:* dantien and see ME page 285.
>
> **illness:** Danburite, Dendritic Chalcedony, Cat's Eye, Golden Danburite, Petrified Wood, Poppy Jasper, Que Sera, Shungite, Trummer Jasper. *Chakra:* earth star, solar plexus, higher heart

Circadian rhythm: Fluorapatite. *Chakra:* dantien, alta major

Circulation: Alabaster, Anglesite, Azurite and Malachite (use as polished stone, make essence by indirect method), Bloodstone, Blue Tiger's Eye, Brazilianite, Brookite, Budd Stone (African Jade), Bustamite, Candle Quartz, Citrine,

Clinohumite, Dendritic Agate, Fiskenaesset Ruby, Fulgarite, Garnet in Quartz, Green Diopside, Howlite, Merlinite, Molybdenite, Morion, Ocean Jasper, Ouro Verde, Pyroxmangite, Rhodochrosite, Riebekite with Sugilite and Bustamite, Rose Quartz, Rosophia, Ruby, Stibnite, Thulite, Trigonic Quartz, Yellow Topaz. *Chakra:* dantien, heart

> **defective:** Blue John, Diamond, Garnet, Merlinite, Ruby, Triplite

> **fortify:** Blue Herkimer with Boulangerite, Pyrope Garnet, Tanzine Aura Quartz

> **peripheral:** Dianite, Ouro Verde, Spangolite

Circulatory:

> **disorders:** Bloodstone, Electric-blue Obsidian, Fulgarite, Hawk's Eye, Hematite, Ruby

> **system:** Amethyst, Bloodstone, Chalcedony, Dendritic Agate, Hematite, Iron Pyrite, Jasper, Magnetite (Lodestone), Red Jasper

Clarity, promote: Adamite, Ammolite, Blue Moonstone, Blue Quartz, Chinese Chromium Quartz, Chinese Red Quartz, Datolite, Dumortierite, Green Ridge Quartz, Holly Agate, Judy's Jasper, Lemurian Seed, Leopardskin Jasper, Limonite, Marcasite, Morion, Pearl Spar Dolomite, Purpurite, Rainforest Jasper, Scapolite, Seriphos Quartz, Silver Leaf Jasper, Realgar and Orpiment, Smoky Candle Quartz, Super 7, Tangerine Sun Aura Quartz, Tugtupite. *Chakra:* third eye, alta major, crown

---

Unless otherwise directed, apply crystal over chakras, organ or site of symptom, wear as jewellery, bathe with or use as crystal essence.

Clearing 'bad vibes': Amazonite, Amber, Amethyst, Aventurine, Black Tourmaline, Chlorite Quartz, Fluorite, Fulgarite, Graphic Smoky Quartz, Iron Pyrite, Kyanite, Lepidolite, Magnetite, Quartz, Selenite, Shieldite, Shungite, Smoky Elestial Quartz, Smoky Quartz, Tantalite, Tektite

Cognitive disorders: Crystal Cap Amethyst and see Mind etc. page 289. *Chakra:* alta major

Compassion for oneself and others: Ajoite, Brandenberg Amethyst, Cobalto Calcite, Erythrite, Gaia Stone, Goethite, Green Diopside, Greenlandite, Green Ridge Quartz, Mangano Vesuvianite, Paraiba Tourmaline, Shaman Quartz, Smoky Cathedral Quartz, Starseed Quartz, Tangerose, Tanzanite, Tugtupite. *Chakra:* heart seed

Concentration, improve: Carnelian, Chrysoberyl, Datolite, Diamond, Fluorite, Goethite, Green Tourmaline, Hematite, Herderite, Jade, Lapis Lazuli, Magnetite, Malachite, Obsidian, Red Jasper, Ruby, Schalenblende. *Chakra:* third eye

Confusion, disperse: Amethyst, Azurite, Bloodstone, Blue Scapolite, Carnelian, Celestial Quartz, Charoite, Crystal Cap Amethyst, Elestial Quartz, Fluorite Gabbro, Hematoid Calcite, Howlite, Kakortokite, Lapis Lazuli, Lepidocrosite, Limonite, Magnetite, Opal, Owyhee Blue Opal, Paraiba Tourmaline, Pietersite, Quartz, Rhodochrosite, Sapphire, Selenite, Sodalite. *Chakra:* between third eye and soma

Connect:

alta major and soma chakra: Andara Glass

earth and soul star chakras: Celestobarite, Orange River Quartz

earth star, base and soul star: Kundalini Quartz, Shungite

earth star, base, heart, crown and soul star: Kakortokite

earth star, base, sacral and stellar gateway: Que Sera

heart seed chakra with soul star: Khutnohorite

heart seed, third eye, soma chakra: Natrolite, Scolecite

heart, soma and soul star chakras: Dianite, Violane

kundalini from crown chakra to higher crown chakras: Amethyst, Amethyst with Hematite, Brandenberg Amethyst, Red Amethyst, Sugilite (Luvulite), Vera Cruz Amethyst

solar plexus, third eye, crown and higher crown chakras with the soul star: Golden Enhydro Herkimer

soma, crown, soul star, stellar gateway chakras and beyond: Fire and Ice, Merkabite Calcite

third eye, crown and soul star chakras: Prophecy Stone

third eye, soma, alta major, crown, stellar gateway and soul star: Afghanite, Anandalite, Auralite 23, Lemurian Seed

third eye, soma and higher crown chakras: Lavender-purple Opal

---

Unless otherwise directed, apply crystal over chakras, organ or site of symptom, wear as jewellery, bathe with or use as crystal essence.

Conscious dreaming: Bowenite (New Jade), Chinese Writing Stone, Lemurian Seed, Owyhee Blue Opal

Contraindications and cautions:

bipolar: avoid Rainbow Mayanite, Red Bushman Quartz, Trigonic Quartz

catharsis, may induce: Barite, Epidote, Hypersthene, Smoky Spirit Quartz, Tugtupite (replace with Quantum Quattro or Smoky Quartz)

delicate/sensitive people, may overstimulate: Rainbow Moonstone, Red Bushman Quartz, Scolecite, Tanzanite, Tremolite

depressed: avoid Granite

dizziness, may cause: Preseli Bluestone (change direction)

during full moon: Blue or Rainbow Moonstone – use Black instead

epilepsy: Dumortierite, Goethite, Zircon

giddiness, remove if causes: Banded Agate

headache and nausea, if causes remove: Hanksite (then place Smoky Quartz on earth star), Preseli Bluestone (or turn the stone)

heart palpitations, if causes remove: Eilat Stone, Malachite

hysterical: Red Bushman Quartz

illusion, may induce: Blue or Rainbow Moonstone

insomnia: Do not wear Herkimer Diamond earrings or place on third eye, avoid Rose Quartz by the bed.

negative energy heightened if worn constantly:

Unless otherwise directed, apply crystal over chakras, organ or site of symptom, wear as jewellery, bathe with or use as crystal essence.

Epidote, Hypersthene

Preseli Bluestone: Do not place in bedroom overnight, turn to align with inherent magnetism.

psychiatric conditions, paranoia or schizophrenia: Do not use crystals unless under the supervision of a qualified crystal healer.

radioactive: Very dark Smoky Quartz, Uranophane

sensitive people: Tanzanite may overstimulate psychic abilities as may Rainbow or Blue Moonstone (use black or pink Moonstone instead).

Tanzanite/Blue Moonstone/Rainbow Moonstone: may create uncontrolled psychic experiences or mental overload or unwanted telepathy

toehold in incarnation: avoid Gabbro with Moonstone, Llanite (Llanoite), Polychrome Jasper. *Chakra:* earth star and soma

toxic, the following crystals may contain traces of toxic mineral although these are bound up within the structure (use polished stone, make crystal essence by indirect method, wash hands after handling):

Actinolite, Adamite, Andaluscite, Ajoite, Alexandrite, Almandine Garnet, Amazonite, Aquamarine, Aragonite, Arsenopyrite, Atacamite, Aurichalcite, Axinite, Azurite, Beryl, Beryllium, Biotite (ferrous), Bixbite, Black Tourmaline, Boji Stones, Bornite, Brazilianite, Brochantite, Bumble Bee Jasper, Cassiterite, Cavansite, Celestite,

Cerussite, Cervanite, Chalcantite, Chalcopyrite (Peacock Ore), Chrysoberyl, Chrysocolla, Chrysotile, Cinnabar, Conichalcite, Copper, Covellite, Crocoite, Cryolite, Cuprite, Diopside, Dioptase, Dumortierite, Emerald, Epidote, Galena, Garnet, Garnierite (Falcondoite), Gem Silica, Germanium, Goshenite, Heliodor, Hessonite Garnet, Hiddenite, Jadeite, Jamesonite, Iolite, Kinoite, Klinoptilolith, Kunzite, Kyanite, Labradorite, Lapis Lazuli, Lazurite, Lepidolite, Magnetite, Malachite, Malacholla, Marcasite, Messina Quartz, Mohawkite, Moldavite, Moonstone, Moqui Balls, Morganite, Orpiment, Pargasite, Piemontite, Pietersite, Plancheite, Prehnite, Psilomelane, Pyrite, Pyromorphite, Quantum Quattro, Que Sera, Realgar, Realgar and Orpiment, Renierite, Rhodolite Garnet, Ruby, Sapphire, Serpentine, Smithsonite, Sodalite, Spessartine Garnet, Sphalerite, Spinel, Spodumene, Staurolite, Stibnite, Sugilite, Sulphur, Sunstone, Tanzanite, Tiffany Stone, Tiger's Eye, Topaz, Torbenite, Tourmaline, Tremolite, Turquoise, Uranophane, Uvarovite Garnet, Valentinite, Vanadinite, Variscite, Vesuvianite, Vivianite, Wavellite, Wulfenite, Zircon, Zoisite

Control freak: Chrysotile, Ice Quartz, Lazulite, Lemurian Aquitane Calcite, Spider Web Obsidian. *Chakra:* dantien

Core:

energy: Erythrite, Lemurian Jade, Menalite, Poppy Jasper, Silver Leaf, Jasper, Smoky Rose Quartz, Trummer Jasper. *Chakra:* dantien

strength/stability: Crinoidal Limestone, Eye of the Storm, Flint, Golden Healer Quartz, Hematite, Mohawkite, Polychrome Jasper

Cosmic anchor: see Anchor page 216

Creativity, improve: Amethyst Herkimer, Bixbite, Blue Quartz, Bushman Quartz, Covellite, Eilat Stone, Girasol, Greenlandite, Icicle Calcite, Quantum Quattro, Rainforest Jasper, Septarian, Seriphos Quartz, Tangerine Sun Aura Quartz, Triplite. *Chakra:* sacral, dantien

– D –

Dark moods, ameliorate: Kunzite, Rutilated Quartz. *Chakra:* solar plexus, third eye

Debility: Black Tourmaline, Fire Agate. *Chakra:* base

Decision making, overcome inability in: Azurite, Green Tourmaline, Rutilated Quartz

Degenerative disease: Ammolite, Brown Jasper, Budd Stone (African Jade), Citrine, Holly Agate, Moonstone, Nuummite, Pearl, Ruby, Scolecite with Natrolite, Stichtite. *Chakra:* dantien, higher heart

Depression: Ajo Blue Calcite, Amber, Amethyst, Ametrine, Apatite, Apophyllite Botswana Agate, Carnelian, Chrysoprase, Citrine, Clinohumite, Dianite, Eisenkiesel, Eudialyte, Flint, Garnet, Golden Healer, Green Ridge Quartz, Hematite, Idocrase, Jade, Jet, Kunzite, Lapis Lazuli, Lepidolite, Lithium Quartz, Macedonian Opal, Maw Sit Sit, Montebrasite, Moss Agate, Orange Kyanite, Pink Sunstone, Porphyrite (Chinese Letter Stone), Purple Tourmaline, Rainbow Goethite, Rutilated Quartz, Siberian Quartz, Sillimanite, Smoky Quartz, Spessartine Garnet, Spider Web Obsidian, Spinel, Staurolite, Sunstone, Tiger's Eye, Tugtupite, Turquoise. *Chakra:* solar plexus. Wear continuously.

Depressive psychosis: Tugtupite. *Chakra:* higher heart (wear continuously, treat under the supervision of a qualified crystal healer).

Detoxification: Amber, Amechlorite, Amethyst,

Unless otherwise directed, apply crystal over chakras, organ or site of symptom, wear as jewellery, bathe with or use as crystal essence.

Anhydrite, Apache Tear, Aventurine, Azurite, Banded Agate, Barite, Bastnasite, Bloodstone, Chalk, Chlorite, Chlorite Quartz, Chrysoprase, Conichalcite, Coprolite, Covellite, Cuprite with Chrysocolla, Dendritic Agate, Diaspore, Emerald, Eye of the Storm, Fire Obsidian, Galena (wash hands after use, make essence by indirect method), Golden Danburite, Golden Healer Quartz, Graphic Smoky Quartz, Green Garnet, Greensand, Halite, Hanksite, Herkimer Diamond, Hypersthene, Iolite, Jade, Jamesonite, Jet, Kambaba Jasper, Larvikite, Malachite, Merlinite, Mica, Obsidian, Ocean Jasper, Orgonite, Phlogopite, Poppy Jasper, Pumice, Quantum Quattro, Que Sera, Rainbow Covellite, Richterite, Ruby, Seraphinite, Shungite, Smoky Elestial Quartz, Smoky Quartz, Smoky Quartz with Aegirine, Stilbite, Sulphur, Sulphur in Quartz, Thunder Egg, Tiger's Eye, Topaz, Tree Agate, Turquoise, Zoisite. *Chakra:* solar plexus, earth star, base

Diabetes/blood sugar imbalances: Angel's Wing Calcite, Astraline, Atlantasite, Bastnasite, Bowenite (New Jade), Chinese Chromium Quartz, Chrome Diopside, Chrysotile in Serpentine, Citrine, Datolite, Diamond (worn at waist, on left side, as close to the pancreas as possible), Emerald, Huebnerite, Jade, Malachite (use as polished stone, make essence by indirect method), Malacholla, Maw Sit Sit, Mtrolite, Owyhee Blue Opal, Pink Opal, Quantum Quattro, Que Sera, Red Jasper, Red Serpentine, Schalenblende, Serpentine, Serpentine in

Obsidian, Shungite, Stichtite, Stichtite with Serpentine, Tugtupite, and see Blood sugar page 224 and Pancreas page 300. *Chakra:* dantien, spleen

Diarrhoea: Green Tourmaline, Lapis Lazuli, Malachite (use as polished stone, make essence by indirect method), Pearl, Quartz, Serpentine

Digestion: Amblygonite, Chrysocolla, Citrine, Coprolite, Covellite, Golden Selenite, Iron Pyrite, Labradorite, Leopardskin Jasper, Limonite, Morion, Mystic Topaz, Obsidian, Ocean Jasper, Peridot, Rhodonite, Sapphire, Shungite, Smithsonite, Snowflake Obsidian, Steatite, Tiger's Eye, Topaz, Yellow Apatite. *Chakra:* solar plexus, dantien

> **calm:** Chrysocolla, Chrysoprase, Green Jasper, Iron Pyrite
>
> **faulty:** Red Tourmaline, Yellow Jasper
>
> **stimulate:** Moss Agate, Red Jade
>
> **strengthen:** Iron Pyrite

Digestive:

> **organs, problems:** Anthrophyllite, Klinoptilolith, Shungite. Place over site.
>
> **organs, strengthen:** Bustamite, Empowerite, Fire Agate, Jasper, Kambaba Jasper, Montebrasite, Pyrite in Quartz, Serpentine in Obsidian, Shungite, Snakeskin Pyrite, Topaz. *Chakra:* dantien, solar plexus
>
> **tract:** Amethyst, Anthrophyllite, Cat's Eye Quartz, Chrysocolla, Crackled Fire Agate, Pink Tourmaline, Serpentine in Obsidian

---

Unless otherwise directed, apply crystal over chakras, organ or site of symptom, wear as jewellery, bathe with or use as crystal essence.

Disconnection from Earth: Flint, Granite, Hematite, Lemurian Jade, Libyan Gold Tektite, Preseli Bluestone, Quartz, Smoky Elestial Quartz, Strontianite, Tektite and see Grounding. *Chakra:* dantien, soma, Gaia gateway

Discontent: Covellite

Dis-ease due to stress: Amechlorite, Basalt, Bird's Eye Jasper, Black Moonstone, Eye of the Storm, Galaxyite, Lemurian Gold Opal, Macedonian Opal, Marble, Orgonite, Richterite, Riebekite with Sugilite and Bustamite, Shungite, Tektite, Tugtupite and see Stress page 320

Disorganisation: Blue Quartz

Distress: Eye of the Storm, Lemurian Gold Opal, Owyhee Blue Opal, Tugtupite. *Chakra:* heart

Dizziness: Aragonite, Candle Quartz, Cathedral Quartz, Dioptase, Eye of the Storm, Flint, Golden Healer Quartz, Hematite, Lapis Lazuli, Mohawkite, Poppy Jasper, Quartz, Richterite, White Sapphire. *Chakra:* dantien, crown, earth star

DNA: Eye of the Storm. *Chakra:* dantien, higher heart

  ancestral: see page 215

  degeneration, reverse: Cavansite, Eye of the Storm, Petrified Wood, Pyrite in Quartz, Snakeskin Pyrite

  mitochondrial: Calcite Fairy Stone, Eye of the Storm, Feather Pyrite, Poppy Jasper, Titanite (Sphene). *Chakra:* dantien

  repair: Brandenberg Amethyst, Eye of the Storm, Rutilated Quartz, Snakeskin Pyrite

---

Unless otherwise directed, apply crystal over chakras, organ or site of symptom, wear as jewellery, bathe with or use as crystal essence.

12 strand: Eye of the Storm, Leopardskin Jasper, Petrified Wood, Quantum Quattro

Dysfunctional patterns, dissolve: Alunite, Arfvedsonite, Celadonite, Dumortierite, Fenster Quartz, Garnet in Quartz, Glendonite, Rainbow Covellite, Scheelite, Stellar Beam Calcite, Spider Web Obsidian

– E –

Ears: Covellite, Eclipse Stone, Goethite, Mystic Topaz, Peanut Wood and see Hearing page 264. *Chakra:* past life, alta major

> **deafness:** Peanut wood
>
> **inner:** Ammolite
>
> **tinnitus:** Ammolite, Black Tourmaline, Dogtooth Calcite, Ocean Jasper, Peanut Wood, Serpentine, Xenotine. *Chakra:* past life, alta major

Earth's chakras, healing: Ammolite, Aragonite, Black Diopside, Black Tourmaline, Blue Sapphire, Brown Aragonite, Bustamite, Cacoxenite, Celestial Quartz, Champagne Aura Quartz, Chlorite Quartz, Desert Rose, Dragon Stone, Eye of the Storm, Feldspar, Flint, Fulgarite, Golden or Tangerine Lemurians, Granite, Greenlandite, Green Ridge Quartz, Kambaba Jasper, Labradorite, Lemurian Jade, Marble, Mohawkite, Monazite, Prehnite, Preseli Bluestone, Quartz, Rhodozite, Scolecite, Selenite, Seriphos Quartz, Smoky Brandenberg, Smoky Elestial, Smoky Quartz, Specular Hematite, Stromatolite, Super 7, Tantalite, Thunder Egg, Torbernite, Witches Finger, Z-stone. *Chakra:* earth star, Gaia gateway. Place in environment.

Egotism, balance: Beryl, Bixbite, Black Onyx, Blue Goldstone, Citrine, Hematoid Calcite, Lepidocrosite, Magnesite, Malachite with Azurite, Mangano Calcite, Morganite, Scheelite, Rainforest Jasper, Rathbunite, Red

Amethyst, Ruby, Sardonyx, Spirit Quartz, Tree Agate. *Chakra:* base, heart

Electrical systems of body, rebalance: Amber, Amblygonite, Cavansite, Galena (wash hands after use, make essence by indirect method), Golden Healer Quartz, Montebrasite, Orgonite, Pollucite, Shiva Lingam, Shungite

Electrolytes, nerve and muscle function: Coral, Malachite, Native Copper, Quartz

Emotional/emotions: *Chakra:* solar plexus, heart

  abuse: Azeztulite with Morganite, Cobalto Calcite, Eilat Stone, Lazurine, Pink Crackle Quartz, Proustite, Tugtupite. *Chakra:* sacral, heart

  alienation: Cassiterite

  angst: Hemimorphite

  attachment: Brandenberg, Drusy Golden Healer, Hemimorphite, Pink Crackle Quartz, Rainbow Mayanite, Tinguaite

  autonomy: Faden Quartz. *Chakra:* dantien

  baggage: Ajoite, Golden Healer Quartz, Rose Elestial Quartz, Tangerose. *Chakra:* solar plexus

  balance: Amblygonite, Dalmatian Stone, Eilat Stone

  black hole: Ajoite, Cobalto Calcite, Quantum Quattro. *Chakra:* higher heart

  blackmail: Tugtupite. *Chakra:* solar plexus

  blockages: Aegirine, Botswana Agate, Bowenite (New Jade), Clinohumite, Cobalto Calcite, Eilat Stone, Green Ridge Quartz, Prehnite with Epidote, Pyrite and

Sphalerite, Quantum Quattro, Rainbow Mayanite, Rhodozite, Tangerose, Tanzine Aura Quartz. *Chakra:* solar plexus

blockages from past lives: Aegirine, Datolite, Dumortierite, Graphic Smoky Quartz (Zebra Stone), Prehnite with Epidote, Pyrite and Sphalerite, Quantum Quattro, Rhodozite, Rose Elestial Quartz, Serpentine in Obsidian, and see Past life healing page 301. *Chakra:* past life

bondage: Ajoite. *Chakra:* solar plexus

bond in relationships, disconnect: Amblygonite, Banded Agate, Brandenberg Amethyst, Flint, Rainbow Mayanite, Shiva Lingam, Stibnite, Tugtupite, Wind Fossil Agate

bond in relationships, heal weak: Dumortierite, Garnet, Green Aventurine, Ice Quartz, Quantum Quattro, Ruby, Rutile, Strawberry Quartz, Vivianite. *Chakra:* heart

burn-out: Cobalto Calcite, Golden Healer Quartz, Lilac Quartz. *Chakra:* heart

catharsis, induce: Barite, Serpentine in Obsidian, Tugtupite

conditioning: Clevelandite, Drusy Golden Healer, Golden Healer Quartz. *Chakra:* solar plexus, third eye

debris: Ajoite, Pink Lemurian Seed, Rainbow Mayanite. *Chakra:* solar plexus

dependency: Cobalto Calcite. *Chakra:* base

dysfunction: Chinese Red Phantom Quartz, Fenster

Quartz, Orange Kyanite. *Chakra:* higher heart

equilibrium: Adamite, Merlinite, Quantum Quattro, Rutile with Hematite, Shungite

exhaustion: Cinnabar in Jasper, Lilac Quartz, Orange River Quartz, Prehnite with Epidote

express: Blue Aragonite

frozen feelings: Clevelandite, Diopside, Eilat Stone, Ice Quartz, Scolecite. *Chakra:* solar plexus, heart, heart seed, higher heart

healing: Garnet in Quartz, Mount Shasta Opal, Tugtupite, Xenotine

hooks, remove: Amblygonite, Drusy Golden Healer, Goethite, Golden Danburite, Klinoptilolith, Novaculite, Nunderite, Nuummite, Orange Kyanite, Pyromorphite, Rainbow Mayanite, Tantalite, Tugtupite. *Chakra:* solar plexus

manipulation: Pink Lemurian Seed, Tantalite. *Chakra:* sacral, solar plexus, third eye

maturation: Alexandrite, Cobalto Calcite

negative, destructive attachments: Ajoite, Drusy Golden Healer, Ilmenite, Pink Lemurian Seed, Rainbow Mayanite, Tantalite, Tinguaite. *Chakra:* base, solar plexus

pain after separation: Aegirine, Eilat Stone, Tugtupite. *Chakra:* higher heart

patterns: Arfvedsonite, Brandenberg Amethyst, Celadonite, Fenster Quartz, Rainbow Covellite, Scheelite. *Chakra:* solar plexus, base

Unless otherwise directed, apply crystal over chakras, organ or site of symptom, wear as jewellery, bathe with or use as crystal essence.

recovery: Empowerite, Eye of the Storm, Lilac Quartz. *Chakra:* higher heart

release: Cobalto Calcite. *Chakra:* solar plexus, base, sacral

restore trust: Clevelandite, Faden Quartz, Xenotine

revitalize: Orange River Quartz, Vivianite

shock: Tantalite, Tugtupite. *Chakra:* heart

shut down, release: Ice Quartz

stability: Mohawkite. *Chakra:* base

stamina: Picrolite

strength: Brazilianite, Mohawkite, Picrolite, Tree Agate. *Chakra:* heart

stress: Cobalto Calcite, Eye of the Storm, Icicle Calcite, Shungite, Tugtupite. *Chakra:* solar plexus

tension: Strawberry Quartz. *Chakra:* solar plexus

toxicity: Ajoite, Arsenopyrite, Banded Agate, Champagne Aura Quartz, Drusy Danburite with Chlorite, Valentinite and Stibnite

trauma: Ajoite, Blue Euclase, Cobalto Calcite, Empowerite, Epidote, Gaia Stone, Graphic Smoky Quartz (Zebra Stone), Holly Agate, Mangano Vesuvianite, Orange River Quartz, Richterite, Tantalite, Tugtupite, Victorite. *Chakra:* solar plexus

turmoil: Cobalto Calcite, Desert Rose. *Chakra:* base

underlying causes of distress: Eye of the Storm, Gaia Stone, Lemurian Gold Opal, Richterite, Riebekite with Sugilite and Bustamite, Smoky Amethyst. *Chakra:* solar plexus, past life

---

Unless otherwise directed, apply crystal over chakras, organ or site of symptom, wear as jewellery, bathe with or use as crystal essence.

wounds: Ajoite, Bustamite, Cassiterite, Cobalto Calcite, Eilat Stone, Gaia Stone, Macedonian Opal, Mookaite Jasper, Orange River Quartz, Piemontite, Rathbunite™, Xenotine. *Chakra:* higher heart

Endocrine system: Adamite, Alexandrite, Amber, Amechlorite, Amethyst, Aquamarine, Azeztulite with Morganite, Black Moonstone, Bloodstone, Blue Quartz, Bustamite, Champagne Aura Quartz, Chrysoberyl, Citrine, Fire Agate, Fire and Ice Quartz, Golden Healer, Golden Topaz, Green Calcite, Green Obsidian, Howlite, Magnetite, Menalite, Pargasite, Pentagonite, Peridot, Picrolite, Pietersite, Pink Heulandite, Pink Tourmaline, Poppy Jasper, Quantum Quattro, Que Sera, Rhodochrosite, Richterite, Ruby Aura Quartz, Seriphos Quartz, Smoky Amethyst, Sodalite, Topaz, Tourmaline, Trummer Jasper, Yellow Jasper. *Chakra:* dantien, higher heart, alta major

Endurance, boost: Chalcedony, Honey Phantom Calcite, Jade, Poppy Jasper, Septarian, Triplite. *Chakra:* base, sacral, dantien

Energetic well-being: Cinnabar Jasper, Fire Agate, Golden Healer Quartz, Jamesonite, Quantum Quattro, Que Sera, Poppy Jasper, Tantalite, Trummer Jasper

Energize chakras: Anandalite, Brandenberg Amethyst, Garnet, Triplite

Energy: Agate, Amber, Amechlorite, Apophyllite, Aragonite, Bloodstone, Blue Goldstone, Calcite, Carnelian, Coral, Danburite, Fire Agate, Garnet, Green

Jasper, Hematite, Jasper, Peridot, Prehnite, Quantum Quattro, Quartz, Que Sera, Rhodochrosite, Ruby, Rutilated Quartz, Strawberry Lemurian, Triplite. *Chakra:* base, sacral, dantien. Or place in environment.

amplify: Garnet, Poppy Jasper, Preseli Bluestone, Ruby Lavender Quartz, Sedona Stone, Triplite. *Chakra:* base, dantien

blockages: Charoite, Danburite, Flint, Fulgarite, Labradorite, Lemurian Quartz, Triplite

depletion, reverse: Eudialyte, Fire Opal, Garnet, Macedonian Opal, Pink Sunstone, Poppy Jasper, Preseli Bluestone, Que Sera, Red Jasper, Ruby Lavender Quartz, Rutilated Quartz, Scheelite, Sedona Stone, Strawberry Lemurian. *Chakra:* dantien

energetic cleanse: Amber, Anandalite, Merlinite

field, strengthen: Garnet, Kunzite, Mohawkite, Poppy Jasper, Preseli Bluestone, Quartz, Ruby Lavender Quartz. *Chakra:* dantien, solar plexus

imbalances: Lepidocrosite

leakage from aura, prevent: Amber, Flint, Garnet, Healer's Gold, Labradorite, Molybdenite in Quartz, Nuummite, Pyrite in Quartz, Rainbow Mayanite, Strawberry Lemurian, Tantalite. *Chakra:* dantien, higher heart

stagnant: Black Tourmaline, Calcite, Clear Topaz, Garnet, Graphic Smoky Quartz, Smoky Elestial Quartz, Smoky Quartz

system: Garnet in Quartz. *Chakra:* dantien

Unless otherwise directed, apply crystal over chakras, organ or site of symptom, wear as jewellery, bathe with or use as crystal essence.

unbalanced field: Amber, Garnet in Quartz, Goldsheen Obsidian, Preseli Bluestone, Ruby in Zoisite

Energy bodies: see The Subtle Energy Bodies and Their Crystals page 209

Energy leakage, prevent: Ajoite with Shattuckite, Flint, Garnet, Green Aventurine, Hematite, Labradorite, Quartz, Shungite. Place over site.

Entities, release from chakras: Petalite, Smoky Amethyst

Entities, remove attached: Drusy Golden Healer, Flint, Klinoptilolith, Larvikite, Nirvana Quartz, Phantom Selenite, Pyromorphite, Rainbow Mayanite, Smoky Amethyst, Stibnite. *Chakra:* sacral, solar plexus, third eye

Etheric bodies/biomagnetic field, realign/strengthen: Anandalite, Angelinite, Astraline, Ethiopian Opal, Golden Healer Quartz, Gold in Quartz, Green Ridge Quartz

Etheric blueprint: see Subtle Energy Bodies page 209

Everyday reality, difficulty in dealing with: Blue Halite, Bornite, Cathedral Quartz, Dumortierite, Lepidocrosite, Marcasite, Neptunite, Pearl Spar Dolomite, Purpurite. *Chakra:* earth star, dantien (or wear continuously)

Exhaustion: Bismuth, Carnelian, Chlorite Quartz, Cinnabar Jasper, Cuprite with Chrysocolla, Epidote, Eye of the Storm, Fire Opal, Garnet, Golden Healer Quartz, Hematite, Lepidolite, Pietersite, Poppy Jasper, Quantum Quattro, Red Jasper, Ruby, Rutilated Quartz, Scheelite, Sulphur, Tiger Iron, Triplite, Turquoise. *Chakra:* base

---

Extraneous thoughts: Fluorite, Paraiba Tourmaline
Extremities, burning: Fluorapatite
Eyes: Biotite, Blue Chalcedony, Cat's Eye Quartz, Cavansite, Covellite, Fenster Quartz, Fluorapatite, Gaia Stone, Galaxyite, Granite, Indicolite Quartz, Lazulite, Malachite, Nuummite, Paraiba Tourmaline, Pink Granite, Rosophia, Schalenblende, Vivianite

> **cooling:** Gaia Stone, Halite, Jamesonite, Paraiba Tourmaline
>
> **optic nerve:** Eudialyte, Kakortokite. *Chakra:* third eye
>
> **retina:** Schalenblende
>
> **soothe:** Blue Chalcedony, Malachite, Paraiba Tourmaline
>
> **strengthen muscles:** Aegirine, Bustamite, Cat's Eye Quartz, Nzuri Moyo, Phlogopite
>
> **tired:** Scapolite
>
> **weak:** Fenster Quartz, Huebnerite, Mystic Topaz

– F –

Fatigue: Amethyst, Ametrine, Bloodstone, Blue Opal, Carnelian, Dendritic Agate, Dioptase, Galena (wash hands after use, make essence by indirect method), Hematite, Iron Pyrite, Red Amethyst, Rose Quartz, Staurolite, Sunstone, Triplite. *Chakra:* dantien

Fear: Blue Quartz, Cacoxenite, Carrolite, Dumortierite, Hackmanite, Icicle Calcite, Leopardskin Jasper, Oceanite, Paraiba Tourmaline, Spectrolite, Tangerose, Tugtupite. *Chakra:* heart, solar plexus

Feet: Bustamite, Petrified Wood, Quantum Quattro, Stromatolite, Zebra Stone

Female reproductive system: Amber, Carnelian, Chrysoprase, Malachite (use as polished stone, make essence by indirect method), Moonstone, Topaz, Unakite, Wulfenite. *Chakra:* sacral, base

Fertility: Basalt, Cinnabar Jasper, Golden Healer Quartz, Menalite, Orange Kyanite

> **increase:** Atacamite, Calcite Fairy Stone, Carnelian, Dragon Stone, Jade, Menalite, Moonstone, Orange Kyanite, Orange Sapphire, Rose Quartz, Ruby in Zoisite, Tree Agate, Triplite, Tugtupite. *Chakra:* sacral, dantien

Fever, lower: Bismuth, Chalcopyrite, Eilat Stone, Gabbro, Honey Opal, Limonite, Macedonian Opal, Pounamu Jade, Pyrite in Magnesite, Sulphur in Quartz, Thompsonite (place stone over site of greatest heat, in front of left ear, on third eye or take as crystal essence)

Forgetfulness: Chlorite Quartz, Emerald, Eye of the Storm, Golden Healer Quartz, Moss Agate, Poppy Jasper, Rhodonite, Sodalite, Tourmaline, Unakite. *Chakra:* third eye

Forgiveness: Diopside, Khutnohorite, Tugtupite. *Chakra:* higher heart

Frigidity/frozen feelings: Poppy Jasper, Red Jasper, Serpentine. *Chakra:* sacral

Frustration, overcome: Chinese Red Quartz, Poppy Jasper, Pyrite in Magnesite. *Chakra:* base, dantien

– G –

Gallbladder: Aegirine, Bytownite, Empowerite, Epidote, Gaspeite, Golden Danburite, Kambaba Jasper, Pyrite in Magnesite, Shungite. *Chakra:* sacral, dantien

Gall, excess: Huebnerite

Genitals: Menalite, Shiva Lingam, Violane. *Chakra:* base

Giddiness: Boji Stones, Emerald, Hematite, Pearl, Quartz, Sodalite. *Chakra:* dantien

Glands: Mookaite Jasper, Paraiba Tourmaline. *Chakra:* dantien, throat

Glandular:

    disturbances: Bastnasite, Mookaite Jasper

    fever: Honey Opal, Paraiba Tourmaline. *Chakra:* throat

    swellings: Agrellite, Anandalite™, Blue Euclase

Grounding kundalini into physical body and physical body to the planet: Ajo Quartz, Amphibole, Auralite 23, Azeztulite, Aztee, Blue Aragonite, Boji Stones, Bronzite, Brown Triplite, Bustamite, Calcite Fairy Stone, Champagne Aura Quartz, Chlorite Quartz, Cloudy Quartz, Dalmatian Stone, Elestial Quartz, Empowerite, Flint, Gabbro, Healer's Gold, Hematite, Hematoid Calcite, Herkimer Diamond, Honey Phantom Quartz, Jasper, Kambaba Jasper, Keyiapo, Lazulite, Lemurian Jade, Lemurian Seed, Leopardskin Serpentine, Libyan Gold Tektite, Limonite, Madagascar Cloudy Quartz, Mahogany Obsidian, Marcasite, Merlinite, Mohawkite, Novaculite, Nunderite, Peanut Wood, Pearl Spar

Dolomite, Petrified Wood, Poppy Jasper, Preseli Bluestone, Purpurite, Pyrite in Magnesite, Quantum Quattro, Red Amethyst, Rutile with Hematite, Schalenblende, Sedona Stone, Serpentine in Obsidian, Smoky Elestial Quartz, Smoky Herkimer, Smoky Quartz, Sodalite, Steatite, Stromatolite, Triplite matrix. *Chakra:* base, earth star, dantien, Gaia gateway

Ground spirit into matter: Aztee, Champagne Aura Quartz, Empowerite, Keyiapo, Khutnohorite, Mohawkite, Peanut Wood, Schalenblende, Serpentine in Obsidian, Steatite. *Chakra:* dantien, soma, Gaia gateway

Guru disconnection: Banded Agate, Rainbow Mayanite. *Chakra:* third eye, soma

– H –

Habits, overcome: Heulandite, Oligocrase, Purpurite. *Chakra:* solar plexus

Hallucinations: Ocean Jasper, Picture Jasper. *Chakra:* third eye, crown

Hands: Stromatolite (hold or wear crystal)

> **cold:** Aragonite and see Raynaud's disease page 310
>
> **swollen:** Trigonic Quartz

Headache: Amber, Amblygonite, Azurite, Blue Sapphire, Bustamite, Cathedral Quartz, Champagne Aura Quartz, Dioptase, Dumortierite, Galena (wash hands after use, make essence by indirect method), Greenlandite, Hematite, Jet, Lapis Lazuli, Magnesite, Quantum Quattro, Quartz, Pyrite in Magnesite, Rhodozite, Rose Quartz, Smoky Quartz, Sugilite, Turquoise. *Chakra:* third eye, alta major

> **arising from:**
>
> > **blocked alta major chakra:** Blue Moonstone, Diaspore, Garnet in Pyroxene, Herderite, Orange Kyanite, Riebekite with Sugilite and Bustamite, and see alta major chakra page 194
> >
> > **blocked kundalini:** see Kundalini crystals page 278
> >
> > **blocked third eye:** Apophyllite, Azurite, Banded Agate, Bytownite, Labradorite
> >
> > **neck tension:** Blue Moonstone, Cathedral Quartz, Magnetite (Lodestone), Quantum Quattro. On base

---

Unless otherwise directed, apply crystal over chakras, organ or site of symptom, wear as jewellery, bathe with or use as crystal essence.

of skull.

Healing crisis: Eye of the Storm, Jade, Quantum Quattro, Que Sera, Smoky Elestial Quartz. *Chakra:* dantien, higher heart

Hearing: Ammolite, Budd Stone (African Jade), Kambaba Jasper, Leopardskin Serpentine, Peanut Wood, Stromatolite and see Ears page 250

> **disorders/tinnitus:** Ammolite, Budd Stone (African Jade), Smoky Amethyst, Snakeskin Agate
>
> **loss:** Kambaba Jasper, Leopardskin Serpentine, Peanut Wood, Stromatolite

Heart (physical): Adamite, Andean Blue Opal, Blue or Green Aventurine, Brandenberg Amethyst, Bustamite, Cacoxenite, Candle Quartz, Fiskenaesset Ruby, Garnet, Garnet in Quartz, Golden Danburite, Green Diopside, Green Heulandite, Green Obsidian, Holly Agate, Khutnohorite, Merlinite, Peridot, Picrolite, Pink or Watermelon Tourmaline, Prasiolite, Quantum Quattro, Rhodochrosite, Rhodonite, Rose Elestial Quartz, Rose Quartz, Rosophia, Sapphire, Tugtupite and see Heart chakra page 199. *Chakra:* heart

> **beat, irregular:** Dumortierite, Jade, Rhodochrosite
>
> **chakra:** see below
>
> **disease:** Carnelian, Eudialyte, Hemimorphite, Morganite, Red Jasper, Rhodochrosite, Rhodonite, Ruby, Smoky Amethyst, Tourmalinated Quartz, Tugtupite
>
> **healer:** Azeztulite with Morganite, Khutnohorite,

Unless otherwise directed, apply crystal over chakras, organ or site of symptom, wear as jewellery, bathe with or use as crystal essence.

Pyroxmangite, Rhodozaz, Roselite, Rosophia

invigorate: Chohua Jasper, Green Garnet, Lemurian Jade

muscle: Kunzite, Septarian

rhythm, disturbed: Brandenberg Amethyst, Calcite, Eye of the Storm, Honey Calcite, Quantum Quattro, Que Sera, Serpentine

strengthen: Calcite, Chohua Jasper, Danburite, Erythrite, Honey Calcite, Lemurian Jade, Pink Lemurian Seed, Rose Quartz, Strawberry Quartz, Tugtupite

trauma, heal: Azeztulite with Morganite, Blue Euclase, Cobalto Calcite, Gaia Stone, Larimar, Mangano Vesuvianite, Oceanite, Peanut Wood, Quantum Quattro, Rose Elestial Quartz, Roselite, Ruby Lavender Quartz, Tantalite, Victorite

unblock: Chohua Jasper, Dioptase, Gaspeite, Green Garnet, Lemurian Jade, Pink Lemurian Seed, Prasiolite, Rose Quartz, Smoky Rose Quartz

Higher crown chakras (stellar gateway, soul star and above): *also see individual entries*

activate: Anandalite, Apophyllite, Azeztulite, Celestite, Green Ridge Quartz, Kunzite, Muscovite, Petalite, Phenacite, Selenite. *Chakras:* soul star, stellar gateway. Place above head.

regulate spin: Amphibole, Anandalite, Angel's Wing Calcite, Brookite, Diaspore (Zultanite), Glendonite, Golden Healer Quartz, Green Ridge Quartz,

Lemurian Aquitane Calcite, Lepidicrosite, Merkabite Calcite™, Novaculite, Paraiba Tourmaline, Titanite (Sphene), Victorite. *Chakras:* soul star, stellar gateway. Place above head and see soul star, stellar gateway.

Higher mind, align: Amethyst Herkimer, Auralite 23, Goethite, Hackmanite, Herderite, Sacred Scribe (Russian Lemurian), Septarian, Sillimanite, Yellow Phantom Quartz. *Chakra:* third eye

Higher self, contact: Amphibole, Anandalite, Anthrophyllite, Bushman Red Cascade Quartz, Cathedral Quartz, Faden Quartz, Fire and Ice Quartz, Golden Healer Quartz, Green Ridge Quartz, Mangano Vesuvianite, Orange River Quartz, Porphyrite (Chinese Letter Stone), Prasiolite, Rosophia, Sugar Blade Quartz, Trigonic Quartz, Ussingite

High vibrational downloads, ground and harmonize: Agnitite™, Ajo Quartz, Anandalite™, Anglesite, Aurichalcite, Aztee, Bismuth, Empowerite, Golden Healer Quartz, Lemurian Gold Opal, Petrified Wood, Phosphosiderite, Rosophia, Ruby Lavender Quartz, Sanda Rosa Azeztulite, Smoky Elestial Quartz, Victorite. *Chakra:* dantien, soma

Hippocampus: Blue Moonstone, Preseli Bluestone. *Chakra:* alta major

Hips, pain: Blue Euclase, Bronzite, Cathedral Quartz, Eilat Stone, Flint, Khutnohorite, Quantum Quattro, Rhodozite, Rutilated Quartz, Serpentine in Obsidian, Smoky Amethyst, Spider Web Obsidian

---

Unless otherwise directed, apply crystal over chakras, organ or site of symptom, wear as jewellery, bathe with or use as crystal essence.

Holes, repair: Amethyst, Anandalite, Flint, Green Tourmaline, Quartz, Rutilated Quartz, Selenite

Homeostasis, maintain: Enstatite and Diopside, Klinoptilolith, Piemontite, Quantum Quattro, Reinerite, Shungite. *Chakra:* dantien

'Hooks', remove: Drusy Golden Healer, Goethite, Klinoptilolith, Nunderite, Orange Kyanite, Pyromorphite, Rainbow Mayanite, Tantalite. *Chakra:* sacral, solar plexus, third eye

Hormones: see also Endocrine system

    boosting: Amechlorite, Amethyst, Cassiterite, Lepidolite, Menalite, Paraiba Tourmaline, Pietersite, Smoky Amethyst. *Chakra:* third eye, higher heart

    imbalances: Amechlorite, Astrophyllite, Black Moonstone, Champagne Aura Quartz, Chinese Chromium Quartz, Chrysoprase, Citrine, Diopside, Hemimorphite, Labradorite, Menalite, Moonstone, Paraiba Tourmaline, Sonora Sunrise, Tanzine Aura Quartz, Tugtupite. *Chakra:* third eye, higher heart

    regulate: Champagne Aura Quartz, Chinese Chromium Quartz, Menalite, Smoky Amethyst, Tugtupite, Watermelon Tourmaline. *Chakra:* third eye, higher heart

Hot flashes/flushes: Crackled Fire Agate, Gabbro, Menalite

Hyperactivity: Black Moonstone, Cerussite, Cumberlandite, Dianite, Fiskenaesset Ruby, Garnet, Green Tourmaline, Lepidocrosite, Montebrasite,

Moonstone, Pearl Spar Dolomite, Yellow Scapolite. *Chakra:* earth star, base, dantien

Hypersensitivity: Dumortierite, Proustite and see Oversensitivity page 299

Hypertension: Apatite

Hyperthyroidism: Atacamite, Cacoxenite, Champagne Aura Quartz, Cryolite, Richterite, Tanzine Aura Quartz. *Chakra:* throat Quartz (or wear continuously)

Hypoglycaemia: Atlantasite, Bowenite (New Jade), Datolite, Maw Sit Sit, Pink Opal, Schalenblende, Stichtite and Serpentine, Tugtupite and see Pancreas page 300. *Chakra:* dantien, spleen

Hypothalamus: Blue Moonstone, Preseli Bluestone, Richterite, Tanzine Aura Quartz

– I –

Illusions:

    assess: Larvikite, Rosophia

    dispel: Adularia, Fairy Wand Quartz, Ilmenite, Kornerupine, Lemurian Seed, Lepidocrosite, Neptunite, Nirvana Quartz, Quartz with Mica, Vivianite

Immune system: Agate, Amechlorite, Ametrine, Anandalite™, Black or Green Tourmaline, Bloodstone, Blue Agate, Brown Jasper, Carnelian, Chevron Amethyst, Chiastolite, Chohua Jasper, Diaspore (Zultanite), Emerald, Fuchsite, Fuchsite with Ruby, Green Calcite, Klinoptilolith, Kunzite, Lapis Lazuli, Lemurian Jade, Lepidolite, Macedonian Green Opal, Malachite (use as polished stone, make essence by indirect method), Mookaite Jasper, Moss Agate, Nzuri Moyo, Ocean Jasper, Paraiba Tourmaline, Pentagonite, Petrified Wood, Preseli Bluestone, Quantum Quattro, Quartz, Que Sera, Reinerite, Richterite, Rosophia, Ruby in Zoisite, Schalenblende, Seriphos Quartz, Shungite, Smithsonite, Smoky Quartz with Aegirine, Super 7, Tangerose, Thunder Egg, Titanite (Sphene), Tourmaline, Turquoise, Winchite, Zoisite. *Chakra:* dantien, higher heart. Place around corners of bed. And see Higher Heart chakra page 200.

Implants, remove: Ajoite, Amechlorite, Cryolite, Drusy Golden Healer, Holly Agate, Ilmenite, Lemurian

Aquitane Calcite, Novaculite, Nuummite, Rainbow Mayanite, Tantalite. *Chakra:* crown

Impotence: Basalt, Bastnasite, Carnelian, Cinnabar Jasper, Garnet, Morganite, Orange Kyanite, Poppy Jasper, Rhodonite, Shiva Lingam, Sodalite, Triplite, Variscite. *Chakra:* base, sacral, dantien

Inadequacy: Eye of the Storm, Poppy Jasper, Pumice. *Chakra:* dantien

Incarnation, ameliorate discomfort in: Ajo Blue Calcite, Celestobarite, Empowerite, Guardian Stone, Keyiapo, Orange Kyanite, Peanut Wood, Pearl Spar Dolomite, Polychrome Jasper, Red Celestial Quartz, Riebekite with Sugilite and Bustamite, Rosophia, Sanda Rosa Azeztulite, Snakeskin Agate, Strontianite, Thompsonite. *Chakra:* soma, dantien and earth star

Indigo/crystal/rainbow/star children: Cat's Eye Quartz, Sanda Rosa Azeztulite, Stichtite, Tremolite, Youngite

Infertility: Banded Agate, Bastnasite, Bixbite, Blue Euclase, Brookite, 'Citrine' Herkimer, Eye of the Storm, Fiskenaesset Ruby, Garnet, Granite, Menalite, Moonstone, Poppy Jasper, Shiva Lingam, Spirit Quartz, Thulite, Triplite, Tugtupite, Zincite. *Chakra:* base and sacral and see Fertility page 259

Inorgasmia: Menalite, Orange Kyanite, Rutile, Shiva Lingam. *Chakra:* base, sacral, dantien

Insomnia: Ajoite, Ajoite with Shattuckite, Amethyst, Bloodstone, Candle Quartz, Celestite, Charoite, Glendonite, Hematite, Howlite, Khutnohorite, Lapis

Lazuli, Lepidolite, Magnetite (Lodestone) (place at head and foot of bed), Moonstone, Mount Shasta Opal, Muscovite, Ocean Jasper, Petrified Wood, Pink Sunstone, Poldervaarite, Rosophia, Selenite, Shungite, Sodalite, Tektite, Topaz, Zoisite. Place by the bed or under the pillow.

> **disturbed sleep patterns:** Khutnohorite, Ocean Jasper, Owyhee Blue Opal, Petrified Wood, Sodalite

> **gastric disturbance causing:** Hackmanite, Khutnohorite, Pyrite in Quartz, Shungite. *Chakra:* solar plexus

Insulin regulation: Astraline, Candle Quartz, Chrysocolla, Malacholla, Maw Sit Sit, Nuummite, Pink Opal, Red Serpentine, Schalenblende, Serpentine in Obsidian, Shungite and see Blood sugar page 224 and Pancreas page 300. *Chakra:* spleen, dantien

> **stabilize:** Ammolite, Septarian. *Chakra:* third eye, crown

Intercellular:

> **blockages:** Fulgarite, Golden Healer Quartz, Gold in Quartz, Plancheite, Pyrite and Sphalerite, Rhodozite, Serpentine in Obsidian

> **structures:** Ajo Blue Calcite, Candle Quartz, Cradle of Life, Golden Healer Quartz, Gold in Quartz, Lemurian Aquitane Calcite, Messina Quartz, Quantum Quattro, Que Sera, Pollucite, Rhodozite, Septarian

Interface:

> **communication with higher beings:** Anandalite,

Angel's Wing Calcite, Lemurian Aquitane Calcite, Mohawkite, Trigonic Amethyst, Trigonic Quartz. *Chakra:* soma, soul star, stellar gateway

self and outside world: Andescine Labradorite, Healer's Gold, Lemurian Jade, Master Shamanite, Mohawkite, Nunderite, Richterite, Serpentine in Obsidian, Spectrolite, Tantalite. *Chakra:* spleen, dantien

Internal organs: Ocean Jasper. *Chakra:* dantien

Intestines: Eclipse Stone, Empowerite, Honey Calcite, Merlinite. *Chakra:* dantien

activate: Basalt

disorders: Bastnasite, Bismuth, Brown Tourmaline, Cryolite, Gaspeite, Halite, Hanksite, Honey Calcite, Scolecite, Septarian. *Chakra:* sacral, dantien

large: Astrophyllite

lower: Rosophia

small: Merlinite, Septarian. *Chakra:* sacral

Intimacy, lack of: Axinite, Datolite, Tugtupite

Intolerance: Pyrite in Magnesite

Introspection: Amphibole Quartz, Steatite. *Chakra:* third eye

Intuitive vision: Amphibole, Anandalite, Auralite 23, Blue Euclase, Blue Selenite Bytownite, Tangerine Aura Quartz, Tanzanite, Tanzine Aura Quartz, and see Third Eye (brow) chakra page 207. *Chakra:* third eye, crown

Involuntary movements, twitches: Fenster Quartz

Irritability: Apatite, Fluorapatite, Jade, Pyrite in

Magnesite, Rhodonite. *Chakra:* base, sacral, dantien

Irritable bowel syndrome (IBS): Amblygonite, Bastnasite, Calcite, Cryolite, Montebrasite, Pumice, Rosophia, Scolecite, Xenotine. *Chakra:* dantien

Irritant filter: Limestone, Pumice, Rhodochrosite. *Chakra:* dantien

– J –

Joints: Azurite, Calcite, Cat's Eye Quartz, Dioptase, Hematite, Magnetite (Lodestone), Messina Quartz, Petrified Wood, Phantom Calcite, Poldervaarite, Rhodonite, Rhodozite

> **calcified:** Calcite, Calcite Fairy Stone, Dinosaur Bone
>
> **flexibility:** Bastnasite, Cavansite, Kimberlite, Peach Selenite, Prehnite with Epidote, Selenite Phantom, Strontianite
>
> **inflamed:** Bloodstone, Blue Chalcedony, Blue Euclase, Blue Lace Agate, Brochantite, Cathedral Quartz, Chalcopyrite, Chrysocolla, Dianite, Diopside, Emerald, Eye of the Storm, Fuchsite, Galena (wash hands after use, make essence by indirect method), Graphic Smoky Quartz, Green Jasper, Hanksite, Hematite, Hematite with Malachite (use as polished stone, make essence by indirect method), Iron Pyrite, Lapis Lazuli, Larimar, Malachite (use as polished stone, make essence by indirect method), Nzuri Moyo, Ocean Jasper, Peach Selenite, Petrified Wood, Quantum Quattro, Rhodonite, Rhodozite, Shungite, Siberian Blue Quartz, Spinel, Sulphur in Quartz, Topaz, Turquoise, Wind Fossil Agate, Zoisite
>
> **mobilize:** Aztee, Calcite Fairy Stone, Fluorite, Nzuri Moyo, Petrified Wood, Prehnite with Epidote, Red Calcite, Strontianite
>
> **pain:** Blue Euclase, Cathedral Quartz, Champagne

Aura Quartz, Eilat Stone, Flint, Khutnohorite, Nzuri Moyo, Quantum Quattro, Rhodozite, Rutilated Quartz, Tantalite

problems: Amber, Apatite, Fluorite, Lepidolite, Obsidian, Sulphur (use as polished crystallized stone, make essence by indirect method)

strengthening: Aragonite, Calcite, Clevelandite, Dinosaur Bone, Tantalite

swollen: Malachite (use as polished stone, make essence by indirect method), Nzuri Moyo, Shungite, Trigonic Quartz, and see inflammation page 274

Journeying: Andean Opal, Aztee, Polychrome Jasper, Preseli Bluestone, Scolecite, Sedona Stone, Serpentine, Serpentine in Obsidian, Shaman Quartz, Stibnite, Titanite (Sphene) and see Shamanic journey page 314

Judgementalism: Green Heulandite, Mohawkite, Tantalite. *Chakra:* dantien

– K –

Karma:

> **burn off:** Chinese Red Quartz and see Past life healing page 301
>
> **of grace, invoke:** Wind Fossil Agate

Karmic: *chakra:* Past Life

> **blueprint:** Cloudy Quartz, Keyiapo, Khutnohorite, Rhodozite, Ruby Lavender Quartz, Sanda Rosa Azeztulite, Scheelite, Titanite (Sphene) and see Subtle Energy Bodies page 209
>
> **cleansing:** Cloudy Quartz, Holly Agate, Lemurian Seed, Wind Fossil Agate
>
> **codependency:** Quantum Quattro, Xenotine
>
> **contracts:** Boli Stone, Gabbro, Leopardskin Jasper, Red Amethyst, Wind Fossil Agate
>
> **debris:** Nuummite, Peach Selenite, Rainbow Mayanite, Smoky Spirit Quartz, Wind Fossil Agate. *Chakra:* past life
>
> **debts:** Holly Agate, Nuummite. *Chakra:* past life
>
> **dis-ease:** Covellite, Isis Calcite, Nuummite and see Past life page 301.. *Chakra:* past life
>
> **emotional healing:** Porphyrite (Chinese Letter Stone), Tangerose
>
> **enmeshment:** Smoky Elestial Quartz
>
> **entanglements:** Flint, Novaculite, Nuummite, Peach Selenite, Rainbow Mayanite
>
> **family burdens:** Mohawkite, Polychrome Jasper,

Unless otherwise directed, apply crystal over chakras, organ or site of symptom, wear as jewellery, bathe with or use as crystal essence.

Tinguaite

healing: Andean Opal, Merlinite, Violane and see Past life healing page 301

wounds: Ajoite, Ajo Quartz, Green Ridge Quartz, Lemurian Seed, Macedonian Opal, Mookaite Jasper, Rathbunite™, Rosophia, Scheelite, Xenotine

Kidneys: Amber, Aquamarine, Bastnasite, Beryl, Black Moonstone, Bloodstone, Blue Quartz, Brookite, Carnelian, Chohua Jasper, Chrysocolla, Citrine, Conichalcite, Diopside, Fiskenaesset Ruby, Gaspeite, Hematite, Heulandite, Jade, Jadeite, Leopardskin Jasper, Libyan Gold Tektite, Muscovite, Nephrite, Nunderite, Nuummite, Orange Calcite, Prehnite with Epidote, Quantum Quattro, Rhodochrosite, Rose or Smoky Quartz, Rosophia, Septarian, Serpentine, Serpentine in Obsidian, Shungite, Sonora Sunrise, Stromatolite, Tanzanite, Topaz. *Chakra:* dantien, solar plexus. Or tape over kidneys.

cleanse: Atacamite, Bloodstone, Brazilianite, Eye of the Storm (Judy's Jasper), Fire and Ice Quartz, Hematite, Jade, Klinoptilolith, Nephrite, Nuummite, Opal, Prehnite with Epidote, Red or Yellow Jasper, Rose Quartz

degeneration: Honey Calcite, Quantum Quattro, Quartz, Red Jasper, Rosophia, Yellow Jasper

detoxify: Amechlorite, Chlorite Quartz, Chohua Jasper, Chrysocolla, Eye of the Storm, Fire and Ice Quartz, Fiskenaesset Ruby, Kambaba Jasper,

Klinoptilolith, Larvikite, Leopardskin Jasper, Nuummite, Quantum Quattro, Pyrite in Magnesite, Rainbow Covellite, Richterite, Seraphinite, Shungite, Smoky Quartz, Smoky Quartz with Aegirine

fortify: Grossular Garnet, Heulandite, Quartz

infection: Citrine, Yellow Zincite

regulating: Carnelian, Muscovite

stimulating: Rhodochrosite, Ruby

stones: Jasper, Magnesite, Rhyolite

underactive: Fire Opal, Prehnite, Rhodochrosite, Ruby

Kundalini crystals: Anandalite, Annabergite, Apatite, Apophyllite, Aquamarine, Atlantasite, Auralite 23, Azeztulite, Bismuth, Black Andradite Garnet (Melanite), Blizzard Stone, Bowenite (New Jade), Brazilianite, Brookite, Carnelian, Chohua Jasper, Cinnabar, Coquimbite, Crocoite, Cryolite, Cuprite, Dioptase, Dragon Stone, Ethiopian Opal, Euclase, Eudialyte, Fire Obsidian, Fire Opal, Firework Obsidian, Fulgarite, Gabbro, Garnet, Garnet in Quartz, Green Ridge Quartz, Growth Interference Quartz, Hemimorphite, Herderite, Himalayan Quartz, Jet, Kundalini Quartz (Congo Citrine), Kunzite, Madagascan Red Celestial Quartz, Magnetite, Moldavite, Nebula Stone, Nirvana Quartz, Orange Creedite, Orange Garnet, Peridot, Phenacite, Poppy Jasper, Purple Herderite, Purple Sapphire, Red Amethyst, Red Ethiopian Opal, Red Jasper, Red Spinel, Red Zincite, Rhodochrosite, Rhodonite, Ruby, Sceptre

Quartz (pair male and female), Scolecite, Sedona Stone, Selenite, Seraphinite, Serpentine, Shiva Lingam, Smoky Quartz, Sonora Sunrise, Spinel, Stichtite, Strontianite, Tibetan Tektite, Tiger's Eye, Topaz, Tremolite, Triplite, Tugtupite, Victorite, Wagnerite

> **alleviate discomfort:** Anandalite, Larimar, Red Amethyst, Serpentine
>
> **balance:** Anandalite, Auralite 23, Celestobarite, Flint, Hematite, Jet, Larimar, Magnetite (Lodestone), Obsidian, Red Jasper, Serpentine, Serpentine in Obsidian, Smoky Quartz, Stichtite with Serpentine, Victorite. *Chakra:* base, knees and earth star
>
> **control rise:** Anandalite, Bismuth, Brown Flash Ethiopian Opal, Jet with Serpentine, Magnetite, Red Amethyst, Serpentine
>
> **Earth's, activate:** Aragonite, Dragon Stone, Fire Obsidian, Kundalini Quartz, Madagascan Red Celestial Quartz, Red Ethiopian Opal, Sedona Stone
>
> **harmonize:** Anandalite, Atlantasite, Larimar, Phenacite, Stichtite with Serpentine
>
> **raise:** Agnitite, Atlantasite, Celestobarite, Ethiopian Opal, Fire Agate, Fire Obsidian, Green Ridge Quartz, Kundalini Quartz, Leopardskin Jasper, Nirvana Quartz, Orange River Quartz, Poppy Jasper, Serpentine, Strawberry Lemurian, Stichtite, Tangerine Aura Quartz, Tangerine Dream Lemurian, Tibetan Tektite. *Chakra:* crown and base
>
> **stimulate rise:** Auralite 23, Azeztulite, Dragon Stone,

Kundalini Quartz, Poppy Jasper, Sedona Stone, Serpentine

– L –

Left-right confusion: Bustamite with Sugilite. *Chakra:* third eye, crown, alta major

Legs: Ametrine, Aquamarine, Bloodstone, Blue Tiger's Eye, Bustamite, Carnelian, Garnet, Hawk's Eye, Jasper, Pietersite, Red Tiger's Eye, Ruby, Smoky Quartz, Tourmaline. *Chakra:* base, sacral

  restless: Hemimorphite

Lethargy: Ametrine, Carnelian, Red Tiger's Eye, Ruby, Tourmaline. *Chakra:* base, sacral

Letting go of past: Axinite, Fenster Quartz, Fulgarite, Green Diopside, Kakortokite, Kimberlite, Lepidocrosite, Nuummite, Paraiba Tourmaline, Pumice, Scheelite, Zircon. *Chakra:* solar plexus, heart, past life

Libido: Crackled Fire Agate, Eudialyte, Kundalini Quartz, Orange Kyanite, Poppy Jasper, Shungite, Sonora Sunrise, Tangerose, Tiffany Stone. *Chakra:* base, sacral

  overactive: Blue Tiger's Eye

  stimulate: Red Tiger's Eye

Life force, increase: Crackled Fire Agate, Libyan Gold Tektite, Moldau Quartz, Poppy Jasper. *Chakra:* higher heart, dantien (or wear continuously) and see Qi page 309

Lightbody: see Subtle Energy Bodies 209

Light-headedness: Celestobarite, Smoky Elestial Quartz, Victorite. *Chakra:* dantien

Limiting patterns of behaviour: Ajoite, Amphibole, Arfvedsonite, Atlantasite, Barite, Botswana Agate,

---

Unless otherwise directed, apply crystal over chakras, organ or site of symptom, wear as jewellery, bathe with or use as crystal essence.

Bronzite, Cassiterite, Celadonite, Chlorite Shaman Quartz, Crackled Fire Agate, Dalmatian Stone, Datolite, Dream Quartz, Dumortierite, Epidote, Garnet in Quartz, Glendonite, Halite, Hanksite, Hematoid Calcite, Honey Phantom Calcite, Indicolite Quartz, Kinoite, Marcasite, Merlinite, Nuummite, Oligocrase, Owyhee Blue Opal, Pearl Spar Dolomite, Porphyrite (Chinese Letter Stone), Quantum Quattro, Rainbow Covellite, Scheelite, Spider Web Obsidian, Stellar Beam Calcite. *Chakra:* base, sacral, dantien, solar plexus, past life

Liver: Amber, Amethyst, Aquamarine, Azurite with Malachite (use as polished stone, make essence by indirect method), Beryl, Black Moonstone, Bloodstone, Blue Holly Agate, Brookite, Carnelian, Charoite, Chrysoprase, Cinnabar in Jasper, Citrine, Danburite, Eilat Stone, Emerald, Empowerite, Epidote, Fluorite, Gaspeite, Gold Calcite, Golden Danburite, Guinea Fowl Jasper, Heulandite, Hiddenite, Huebnerite, Labradorite, Lazulite, Lepidocrosite, Limonite, Orange River Quartz, Pietersite, Poppy Jasper, Red Amethyst, Red Jasper, Rhodonite, Rose Quartz, Ruby, Shungite, Tiger's Eye, Topaz, Tugtupite, Yellow Fluorite, Yellow Jasper, Yellow Labradorite. *Chakra:* dantien

> **blockages:** Bastnasite, Fulgarite, Gaspeite, Holly Agate, Orange Kyanite, Poppy Jasper, Red Jasper, Red Tourmaline, Rhodozite, Thunder Egg
>
> **blood flow:** Mookaite Jasper
>
> **cleanse:** Charoite, Crystal Cap Amethyst, Gaspeite,

Klinoptilolith, Peridot, Ruby

depletion: Holly Agate, Macedonian Opal, Tugtupite

detoxifying: Amechlorite, Bastnasite, Biotite, Chlorite Quartz, Eye of the Storm, Gaspeite, Kambaba Jasper, Klinoptilolith, Larvikite, Malachite (use as polished stone, make essence by indirect method), Mtrolite, Pyrite in Magnesite, Rainbow Covellite, Richterite, Seraphinite, Shungite, Smoky Quartz with Aegirine, Thunder Egg

stimulate: Amethyst, Azurite, Emerald, Poppy Jasper, Schalenblende, Silver Leaf Jasper, Tantalite, Thunder Egg, Tugtupite, Zircon

Lungs: Adamite, Amber, Amethyst, Ammolite, Andean Blue Opal, Atlantasite, Aventurine, Beryl, Blue Aragonite, Blue Quartz, Botswana Agate, Bustamite, Cacoxenite, Catlinite, Charoite, Chrysocolla, Diopside, Dioptase, Emerald, Fluorapatite, Fluorite, Graphic Smoky Quartz (Zebra Stone), Greenlandite, Hiddenite, Kambaba Jasper, Kunzite, Lapis Lazuli, Morganite, Peridot, Petalite, Petrified Wood, Pink Tourmaline, Prehnite, Prehnite with Epidote, Pyrite in Quartz, Quantum Quattro, Rhodochrosite, Rose Quartz, Sardonyx, Scheelite, Scolecite, Serpentine, Serpentine in Obsidian, Smoky Amethyst, Sodalite, Sonora Sunrise, Stromatolite, Tremolite, Turquoise, Valentinite and Stibnite, Watermelon Tourmaline. *Chakra:* dantien, higher heart

congested: Jade, Kambaba Jasper, Moss Agate, Quantum Quattro, Shungite, Stromatolite, Vanadinite

(make essence by indirect method)

difficulty in breathing: Anthrophyllite, Apophyllite, Chrysocolla, Green Siberian Quartz, Kambaba Jasper, Quantum Quattro, Riebekite with Sugilite and Bustamite, Stromatolite, Tremolite and see Breathlessness page 228

fluid in: Amber, Diamond, Hackmanite, Halite, Hanksite, Ocean Jasper, Scheelite, Smoky Amethyst, Yellow Sapphire, Zircon

Lupus: Chinese Red Quartz, Eudialyte

Lymph: Bloodstone, Chalcedony, Chrysoprase, Moonstone, Shungite, Trigonic Quartz

Lymphatic system: Agate, Anglesite, Bastnasite, Blue Chalcedony, Chlorite Quartz, Eye of the Storm (Judy's Jasper), Graphic Smoky Quartz, Hackmanite, Lazulite, Moonstone, Moss Agate, Ocean Blue Jasper, Scheelite, Shungite, Tourmaline, Trigonic Quartz, Zebra Stone. *Chakra:* dantien, higher heart

cleansing: Agate, Bastnasite, Chlorite Quartz, Crystal Cap Amethyst, Feather Pyrite, Ocean Jasper, Rose Quartz, Shungite, Sodalite, Sugilite, Yellow Apatite

infections: Blue Lace Agate, Shungite

stimulating: Bloodstone, Blue Chalcedony, Ocean Jasper, Oligocrase

swellings: Agrellite, Anandalite™, Blue Euclase, Crystal Cap Amethyst, Jet

– M –

ME: Ametrine, Bismuth, Chinese Red Quartz, Chrysotile in Serpentine, Eye of the Storm, Petrified Wood, Quantum Quattro, Que Sera, Ruby, Shungite, Tourmaline. *Chakra:* dantien

Meditative states, enter easily: Anandalite, Blue Selenite, Bytownite, Golden Azeztulite, Lemurian Seed, Pink Petalite. *Chakra:* third eye, crown

Memory, improve: Amber, Amethyst, Barite, Coprolite, Emerald, Fluorite, Hematoid Calcite, Herderite, Klinoptilolith, Marcasite, Moss Agate, Opal, Phantom Calcite, Pyrite and Sphalerite, Pyrolusite, Rhodonite, Unakite, Vivianite. *Chakra:* third eye, crown

Meniere's disease: Ammolite, Dioptase, Quantum Quattro. Tape behind affected ear.

Menopause: Black Moonstone, Blue Euclase, Eclipse Stone, Lodolite, Menalite, Peach Selenite

Menstrual:

    cramps: Bastnasite, Cat's Eye Quartz, Eilat Stone, Menalite, Orange Moss Agate, Serpentine in Obsidian, Shiva Lingam, Tugtupite. *Chakra:* sacral, base

    cycle, regulate: Menalite, Tugtupite. *Chakra:* sacral, base

Menstruation: Menalite, Tugtupite

    irregular: Menalite, Tugtupite. *Chakra:* sacral, base

Mental:

    agitation: Eye of the Storm, Strawberry Quartz,

Unless otherwise directed, apply crystal over chakras, organ or site of symptom, wear as jewellery, bathe with or use as crystal essence.

Youngite

blockages: Molybdenite, Rhodozite

breakdown: Molybdenite, Novaculite, Quantum Quattro, Youngite. *Chakra:* third eye, crown

clarity: Holly Agate, Merkabite Calcite, Moldau Quartz, Poldervaarite, Realgar and Orpiment, Sacred Scribe, Star Hollandite, Thompsonite

cleansing: Black Kyanite, Blue Quartz, Hungarian Quartz

combine heart and mind: Adamite, Auralite 23

conditioning, rigid: Drusy Golden Healer, Pholocomite, Rainbow Covellite, and negative thought patterns 289. *Chakra:* third eye, crown

confusion: Aegirine, Blue Halite, Blue Quartz, Hematoid Calcite, Limonite, Pholocomite, Poldervaarite, Richterite

detox: Amechlorite, Banded Agate, Drusy Quartz on Sphalerite, Eye of the Storm, Larvikite, Pyrite in Magnesite, Rainbow Covellite, Richterite, Shungite, Smoky Quartz with Aegirine, Spirit Quartz, Tantalite

dexterity/flexibility, improve: Brucite, Bushman Quartz, Coprolite, Green Ridge Quartz, Kimberlite, Limonite, Molybdenite, Seriphos Quartz, Tiffany Stone, Titanite (Sphene). *Chakra:* third eye, crown

dysfunction: Alunite, Star Hollandite, Titanite (Sphene)

exhaustion: Cinnabar in Jasper, Marcasite, Spectrolite

focus: Sacred Scribe (Russian Lemurian)

Unless otherwise directed, apply crystal over chakras, organ or site of symptom, wear as jewellery, bathe with or use as crystal essence.

harmony: Auralite 23, Bytownite (Yellow Labradorite), Fluorite. *Chakra:* third eye

implants: Amechlorite, Blue Halite, Brandenberg, Cryolite, Drusy Golden Healer, Holly Agate, Ilmenite, Lemurian Aquitane Calcite, Limonite, Novaculite, Nuummite, Pholocomite, Tantalite

influences, detach: Flint, Jasper, Kunzite, Selenite

sabotage: Agrellite, Amphibole, Lemurian Aquitane Calcite, Mohawkite, Paraiba Tourmaline, Tantalite, Yellow Scapolite

strength: Plancheite

upheaval: Guinea Fowl Jasper

Meridians:

blocked: Apricot Quartz, Feather Pyrite, Orange Kyanite, Orange River, Polychrome Jasper, Pyrite in Quartz, Que Sera, Shiva Lingam, Snakeskin Pyrite, Spider Web Obsidian, Strawberry Lemurian. *Chakra:* dantien

harmonize planetary: Dragon Stone, Ethiopian Opal, Feather Pyrite, Mohawkite, Monazite, Polychrome Jasper, Que Sera, Spider Web Obsidian, Star Hollandite, Terraluminite

re-align personal: Chrysotile in Serpentine, Feather Pyrite, Lemurian Seed, Orange River Quartz, Pink Lazurine, Polychrome Jasper, Terraluminite. *Chakra:* dantien

stimulate: Pyrite in Magnesite, Pyrite in Quartz, Que Sera, Shiva Lingam, Spider Web Obsidian. *Chakra:*

dantien

Metabolic:

imbalances: Amazonite, Amechlorite, Azurite with Malachite and Chrysocolla (use as polished stone, make essence by indirect method), Blue Opal, Bornite, Champagne Aura Quartz, Chrysocolla, Diamond, Galaxyite, Garnet, Golden Azeztulite, Golden Danburite, Golden Herkimer, Hackmanite, Healer's Gold, Herkimer Diamond, Khutnohorite, Labradorite, Lemurian Jade, Mangano Vesuvianite, Peridot, Quantum Quattro, Que Sera, Shungite, Sonora Sunrise, Tantalite, Tanzine Aura Quartz, Tugtupite, Watermelon Tourmaline, Winchite. *Chakra:* dantien, third eye

stimulate processes: Apatite, Blue Tiger's Eye, Garnet, Hawk's Eye, Red Carnelian, Smoky Amethyst, Tugtupite. *Chakra:* third eye and dantien

syndrome: Amechlorite, Anandalite, Andara Glass, Galaxyite, Klinoptilolith, Quantum Quattro, Que Sera, Richterite, Scheelite, Shungite, Tanzine Aura Quartz, Winchite

system: Amechlorite, Amethyst, Bloodstone, Carnelian, Champagne Aura Quartz, Hackmanite, Labradorite, Piemontite, Smoky Amethyst, Smoky Quartz with Aegirine, Sodalite, Tantalite, Winchite

Metabolism: Amazonite, Amechlorite, Ametrine, Bloodstone, Chrysoprase, Dendritic Agate, Fossilised Wood, Galaxyite, Garnet, Garnet in Pyroxene,

Hackmanite, Klinoptilolith, Labradorite, Piemontite, Pyrite in Magnesite, Quantum Quattro, Que Sera, Ruby, Serpentine, Shungite, Sodalite, Tourmaline, Turquoise, Tree Agate, Tugtupite, Winchite. *Chakra:* dantien

>   **regulate:** Pearl Spa Dolomite

>   **stimulate:** Amethyst, Garnet, Pyrolusite, Sodalite, Tanzine Aura Quartz. *Chakra:* dantien, higher heart

Miasms: Crinoidal Limestone, Flint, Golden Danburite, Kambaba Jasper, Nuummite, Quantum Quattro, Stromatolite. *Chakra:* earth star, base, past life

Migraine: Amethyst, Aventurine, Azurite, Cathedral Quartz, Dioptase, Eye of the Storm (Judy's Jasper), Iolite, Jet, Lapis Lazuli, Magnesite, Pearl, Rhodochrosite, Rose Quartz, Sodalite, Sugilite, Topaz. *Chakra:* third eye, crown, past life

Mind: and see Mental page 285. *Chakra:* third eye, crown

>   **butterfly:** Auralite 23, Calcite, Fluorite, Tantalite

>   **chatter, switch off:** Auralite 23, Bytownite, Rhodozite, Rhomboid Selenite, Richterite, Scheelite and see Over-thinking page 299

>   **control:** Cryolite, Drusy Golden Healer, Pholocomite, Thunder Egg

>   **malicious thoughts, release:** Hemimorphite, Pholocomite, Scolecite

>   **negative thought patterns:** Amphibole, Arfvedsonite, Celadonite, Dumortierite, Nuummite, Owyhee Blue Opal, Rainbow Covellite, Scheelite, Scolecite

Misfit: Tremolite. *Chakra:* base, dantien

Unless otherwise directed, apply crystal over chakras, organ or site of symptom, wear as jewellery, bathe with or use as crystal essence.

Misogyny: Zircon

Mood swings: Amazonite, Eye of the Storm (Judy's Jasper), Kunzite, Serpentine, Turquoise and see Bipolar page 222

Motor dysfunction: Axinite, Basalt, Bustamite, Cat's Eye Quartz, Cumberlandite, Golden Danburite, Klinoptilolith, Kyanite, Peanut Wood, Quartz with Epidote, Scolecite and Natrolite, Sugilite

Motor nerves: Bustamite, Cat's Eye Quartz, Golden Coracalcite, Scheelite

Mouth: Covellite

Mucus membranes: Conichalcite, Hanksite, Oregon Opal, Richterite

Multidimensional:

cellular healing: Ajo Blue Calcite, Ajo Quartz, Anandalite™, Annabergite, Brandenberg Amethyst, Crystal Cap Amethyst, Elestial Quartz, Eudialyte, Fire and Ice Quartz, Fiskenaesset Ruby, Golden Coracalcite, Golden Healer Quartz, Mangano Vesuvianite, Messina Quartz, Pollucite, Que Sera, Rhodozite, Ruby Lavender Quartz

connections: Ajoite, Anandalite™, Angelinite, Astraline, Azotic Topaz, Brandenberg Amethyst, Crystal Cap Amethyst, Crystalline Kyanite, Galaxyite, Hemimorphite, Lemurian Seed, Merlinite, Molybdenite in Quartz, Mystic Topaz, Natrolite, Nirvana Quartz, Sanda Rosa Azeztulite, Satyamani and Satyaloka Quartz, Spirit Quartz, Stellar Beam

Calcite, Tiffany Stone

healing: Ajo Quartz, Anandalite™, Banded Agate, Celestobarite, Eudialyte, Fiskenaesset Ruby, Halite, Hanksite, Icicle Calcite, Kakortokite, Lemurian Seed, Lilac Quartz, Phantom Quartz, Que Sera, Rutile with Hematite, Sanda Rosa Azeztulite, Satyamani and Satyaloka Quartz, Shaman Quartz, Sichuan Quartz, Spirit Quartz, Tangerine Dream Lemurian, Trigonic Quartz

self: Crystal Cap Amethyst, Herderite, Natrolite, Trigonic Quartz

soul work: Anandalite™, Brandenberg Amethyst, Fenster Quartz, Porphyrite (Chinese Letter Stone), Sugar Blade Quartz, Tanzine Aura Quartz, Trigonic Quartz

travel: Afghanite, Anandalite™, Auralite 23, Aztee, Banded Agate, Blue Moonstone, Brandenberg Amethyst, Celestobarite, Golden Selenite, Kinoite, Novaculite, Nunderite, Orange Creedite, Owyhee Blue Opal, Phantom Quartz, Polychrome Jasper, Preseli Bluestone, Rainbow Moonstone, Sedona Stone, Shaman Quartz, Spectrolite, Spirit Quartz, Tanzanite, Thunder Egg, Titanite (Sphene), Trigonic Quartz, Ussingite, Vivianite, Youngite

Multiple personality disorder: Bastnasite, Brucite

Muscles: Bismuth, Black Kyanite, Cat's Eye Quartz, Hematite, Jadeite, Nzuri Moyo, Petrified Wood, Phlogopite, Rhodonite, Scheelite, Titanite (Sphene)

Unless otherwise directed, apply crystal over chakras, organ or site of symptom, wear as jewellery, bathe with or use as crystal essence.

cramps: Apache Tear, Bastnasite, Cat's Eye Quartz, Celestite, Infinite Stone, Larimar, Magnesite, Magnetite (Lodestone), Orange Moss Agate, Quantum Quattro, Serpentine in Obsidian, Smithsonite, Strontianite and see page 296

disorders: Diopside, Kyanite, Peridot, Petalite, Rosophia

dystrophy: Rosophia, Scolecite and Natrolite

flexibility/pain: Aegirine, Blue Euclase, Cathedral Quartz, Cumberlandite, Eilat Stone, Flint, Kimberlite, Rhodozite, Rosophia, Rutilated Quartz, Wind Fossil Agate

spasm: Amazonite, Apache Tear, Azurite with Malachite (use as polished stone, make essence by indirect method), Bornite, Chrysocolla, Diopside, Fuchsite, Magnetite (Lodestone), Malacholla, Petalite, Phlogopite, Pyrite in Magnesite, Red Tourmaline, Strontianite and see Spasms page 317

strengthen: Aegirine, Apatite, Bismuth, Bustamite, Fluorite, Jadeite, Peridot, Tourmaline

swelling: Anandalite™, Andean Blue Opal, Blue Euclase, Brochantite

tension: Basalt, Blue Aragonite, Blue Euclase, Champagne Aura Quartz

tissue: Aventurine, Danburite, Desert Rose, Khutnohorite, Magnetite (Lodestone), Phlogopite, Sonora Sunrise

tone: Fluorite, Peridot, Tourmaline

Unless otherwise directed, apply crystal over chakras, organ or site of symptom, wear as jewellery, bathe with or use as crystal essence.

torn: Creedite, Diaspore (Zultanite), Nzuri Moyo, Tantalite

weak: Rhyolite, Tiger Iron

Muscular-skeletal system inflexibility: Coprolite, Cumberlandite, Fuchsite, Jade, Kimberlite, Limonite, Magnesite, Quantum Quattro, Rosophia, Steatite, Stromatolite

– N –

Nausea: Brown Agate, Dioptase, Emerald, Fuchsite, Green Jasper, Red Aventurine, Sapphire

Necessary change, accept: Axinite, Eclipse Stone, Ethiopian Opal, Luxullianite, Nunderite, Snakeskin Pyrite. *Chakra:* dantien

Neck: Blue Siberian Quartz. *Chakra:* throat

> **tension:** Alexandrite, Blue Moonstone, Blue Siberian Quartz, Rainbow Moonstone

Negative:

> **energy, dispel:** Black Kyanite, Guardian Stone, Hypersthene, Klinoptilolith, Nuummite, Smoky Elestial Quartz, Smoky Herkimer, Tantalite. *Chakra:* throat, earth star
>
> **karma:** Smoky Elestial Quartz and see Past life page 301. *Chakra:* past life

Negativity, dispel: Nuummite, Smoky Elestial Quartz, Tantalite. *Chakra:* earth star

Nerves: Bronzite, Cat's Eye Quartz, Cryolite, Dalmatian Stone, Golden Coracalcite, Merlinite, Nuummite, Phlogopite, Scheelite, Smoky Amethyst, Stichtite, Tanzanite

> **calming:** Eudialyte, Jamesonite
>
> **endings:** Guinea Fowl Jasper, Tinguaite
>
> **motor:** Bustamite, Cat's Eye Quartz
>
> **optic:** see Eyes page 258
>
> **pain relief:** Blue Euclase, Flint, Nuummite,

Rhodozite, Rutilated Quartz, Wind Fossil Agate

regenerating: Natrolite with Scolecite

spinal: Tinguaite

strengthen: Banded Agate, Drusy Quartz on Sphalerite, Mystic Topaz, Nuummite

Nervous:

autonomic system: Anglesite, Aventurine, Barite, Datolite, Dendritic Chalcedony, Golden Coracalcite, Kambaba Jasper, Merlinite, Phantom Calcite, Stichtite, Stromatolite, White Heulandite. *Chakra:* dantien

disorders: Natrolite with Scolecite

exhaustion: Cinnabar in Jasper, Eudialyte

stress: Auralite 23, Eudialyte, Eye of the Storm, Larvikite, Merlinite, Riebekite with Sugilite and Bustamite, Shungite

sympathetic: Cumberlandite. *Chakra:* dantien

system: Aegirine, Alexandrite, Anglesite, Astrophyllite, Azeztulite with Morganite, Banded Agate, Datolite, Dendritic Chalcedony, Epidote, Eudialyte, Greenlandite, Kakortokite, Merlinite, Natrolite, Petrified Wood, Prehnite with Epidote, Stichtite, Stichtite and Serpentine, White Heulandite

tension: Larvikite, Merlinite

Nervousness: Eudialyte

Neural:

fibres: Feather Pyrite, Pyrite and Sphalerite, Scolecite. *Chakra:* dantien

pathways: Golden Coracalcite, Larvikite, Merlinite,

Mystic Merlinite, Natrolite, Phantom Calcite, Scolecite, Stichtite, Tree Agate

transmission: Anglesite, Larvikite, Natrolite, Scolecite, Tremolite

Neurological tissue: Alexandrite, Golden Coracalcite, Natrolite, Phlogopite, Scolecite and see Nerves above

Neurosis: Greenlandite. *Chakra:* solar plexus

Neurotic patterns: Arfvedsonite, Celadonite, Greenlandite, Porphyrite (Chinese Letter Stone), Rainbow Covellite, Scheelite. *Chakra:* solar plexus

Neurotransmitters: Anglesite, Crystal Cap Amethyst, Golden Coracalcite, Kambaba Jasper, Khutnohorite, Ocean Blue Jasper, Phantom Calcite, Que Sera, Scolecite, Shungite, Sodalite, Stromatolite, Tremolite. *Chakra:* alta major (base of skull)

Night:

> **blindness:** Blue Chalcedony, Golden Herkimer, Morion, Quantum Quattro, Sichuan Quartz, Tanzine Aura Quartz, Vivianite
>
> **cramps/twitches:** Blue or White Aragonite, Cat's Eye Quartz, Orange Moss Agate, Pearl Spar Dolomite, Serpentine in Obsidian
>
> **sweats:** Blue Quartz, Indicolite Quartz, Menalite
>
> **terrors:** Diaspore, Pearl Spar Dolomite, Smoky Amethyst, Smoky Elestial Quartz, Tremolite

Nightmares: Amethyst, Celestite, Chrysoprase, Dalmatian Stone, Diaspore, Hematite, Jet, Mangano Calcite, Pearl Spar Dolomite, Prehnite, Rose Quartz,

Ruby, Smoky Quartz, Sodalite, Spirit Quartz, Tremolite, Turquoise. Place under the pillow or around the bed.

Nose: Covellite, Eclipse Stone, Goethite

   bleed: Hausmanite

Nurturing, lack of: Amblygonite, Bornite on Silver, Calcite Fairy Stone, Clevelandite, Cobalto Calcite, Drusy Blue Quartz, Flint, Lazurine, Menalite, Mount Shasta Opal, Ocean Jasper, Prasiolite, Ruby Lavender Quartz, Septarian, Super 7, Tree Agate, Tugtupite. *Chakra:* higher heart, base

– O –

Obsession: Amethyst, Ammolite, Auralite 23, Barite, Bytownite, Fenster Quartz, Golden Selenite, Novaculite, Ocean Jasper, Red Amethyst, Spirit Quartz, Tantalite, Vera Cruz Amethyst. *Chakra:* dantien, solar plexus, third eye

Obsessive behaviour: Ocean Jasper, Smoky Rose Quartz, Tantalite

Obsessive-compulsive disorder: Amethyst Herkimer, Fenster Quartz, Flint, Novaculite, Tantalite

Obsessive thoughts: Ammolite, Auralite 23, Barite, Bytownite, Scolecite, Spirit Quartz, Tantalite. *Chakra:* third eye, crown

Open and align all chakras: Anandalite, Carnelian, Fire Agate, Green Ridge Quartz, Jadeite, Kyanite, Pink Tourmaline and see Chakras page 233

Ovaries: Menalite, Ocean Jasper, Schalenblende. *Chakra:* sacral

Over:

> **active:** Poppy Jasper
>
> **attachment:** Drusy Golden Healer, Rainbow Mayanite, Tantalite, Tinguaite. *Chakra:* solar plexus
>
> **defended:** Honey Opal
>
> **dependent:** Ussingite
>
> **eating:** Crystal Cap Amethyst, Epidote. *Chakra:* base, dantien
>
> **excitability:** Dumortierite, Fiskenaesset Ruby

Unless otherwise directed, apply crystal over chakras, organ or site of symptom, wear as jewellery, bathe with or use as crystal essence.

load: Diopside

reaction: Paraiba Tourmaline

sensitive: Paraiba Tourmaline, Proustite, Riebekite with Sugilite and Bustamite, Scolecite, Shungite, Tremolite. *Chakra:* solar plexus

stimulated: Poppy Jasper

thinking: Auralite 23, Bytownite, Creedite, Dalmatian Stone, Rhomboid Selenite. *Chakra:* third eye

weight: Epidote, Ethiopian Opal, Hemimorphite, Heulandite, Petrified Wood

whelm: Diopside. *Chakra:* solar plexus

work: Prehnite with Epidote, Tanzanite

Overactive mind: Amethyst, Auralite 23, Blue Selenite, Bytownite (Yellow Labradorite), Crystal Cap Amethyst, Rhodozite, Sodalite, Spectrolite. *Chakra:* third eye

Oversensitivity to:

cold: Barite

pressure: Avalonite

temperature changes: Barite, Dinosaur Bone, Luxullianite, Pietersite

weather: Avalonite, Barite, Golden Pietersite

Ovulation pain: Blue Euclase, Crystalline Kyanite, Flint, Menalite, Quantum Quattro, Rhodozite, Rutilated Quartz

Oxygen, malabsorption: Azotic Topaz, Banded Agate, Chinese Red Quartz, Goethite, Kambaba Jasper, Merlinite, Molybdenite, Pyrite in Magnesite, Pyrite in Quartz, Reinerite, Sonora Sunrise, Stromatolite. *Chakra:* dantien. Or place over heart and lungs.

Unless otherwise directed, apply crystal over chakras, organ or site of symptom, wear as jewellery, bathe with or use as crystal essence.

– P –

Painful feelings, assimilate: Khutnohorite, Tugtupite. *Chakra:* heart

Pain relief: Amber, Amethyst, Aragonite, Boji Stones, Cathedral Quartz, Celestite, Dendritic Agate, Fluorite, Hematite, Infinite Stone, Lapis Lazuli, Larimar, Magnetite (Lodestone), Mahogany Obsidian, Malachite (use as polished stone, make essence by indirect method), Quartz, Rose Quartz, Rutilated Quartz, Seraphinite, Smoky Quartz, Sugilite, Tourmaline

Palpitations: Amber, Danburite, Dumortierite, Eye of the Storm, Garnet, Honey Calcite, Rose Quartz, Tugtupite. *Chakra:* dantien and heart

Pancreas: Amber, Astraline, Bloodstone, Blue Lace Agate, Brochantite, Bustamite, Carnelian, Charoite, Chinese Chromium Quartz, Chrysocolla, Citrine, Green Calcite, Huebnerite, Jasper, Leopardskin Jasper, Malachite (use as polished stone, make essence by indirect method), Maw Sit Sit, Moonstone, Pink Opal, Pink Tourmaline, Quantum Quattro, Red Tourmaline, Richterite, Schalenblende, Septarian, Serpentine in Obsidian, Shungite, Smoky Quartz, Tanzine Aura Quartz, Topaz, Tugtupite. *Chakra:* spleen, dantien

Pancreatic secretions: Astraline, Bustamite Muscovite, Malachite (use as polished stone, make essence by indirect method). *Chakra:* spleen, solar plexus, base and see Blood sugar page 224

Panic attacks: Amethyst, Blue-green Smithsonite, Dumortierite, Eye of the Storm, Girasol, Green Phantom Quartz, Green Tourmaline, Kunzite, Serpentine in Obsidian, Tremolite, Turquoise. *Chakra:* heart, higher heart, solar plexus. Keep in pocket and hold when required.

Parathyroid: Blue Siberian Quartz, Cacoxenite, Champagne Aura Quartz, Chrysotile, Chrysotile in Serpentine, Cumberlandite, Kyanite, Leopardskin Jasper, Malachite (use as polished stone, make essence by indirect method), Richterite, Tanzine Aura Quartz. *Chakra:* throat

Parkinson's disease: Anthrophyllite, Black Moonstone, Diaspore, Eudialyte, Kambaba Jasper, Nuummite, Owyhee Blue Opal, Stichtite, Stichtite and Serpentine, Stromatolite. *Chakra:* dantien

Past life chakra issues:

    abandonment: Pink Tourmaline, Rhodonite. *Chakra:* past life, heart

    access: Dumortierite, Preseli Bluestone, Variscite, Wulfenite. *Chakra:* past life, third eye

    addiction, causes of: Iolite. *Chakra:* past life, base

    Akashic Record, read: Blue Aventurine, Brandenberg Amethyst, Cathedral Quartz, Optical Calcite, Prehnite, Tanzanite, Tibetan Black Spot Quartz, Trigonic Quartz. *Chakra:* past life, third eye, crown

    betrayal: Rhodonite. *Chakra:* past life, heart

    blockages from past lives: Lepidolite. *Chakra:* past life

broken heart: Rose Quartz. *Chakra:* past life, heart

chastity vows: Okenite. *Chakra*: past life, base, sacral

cleansing: Danburite. *Chakra:* past life

curses:

>**break:** Shattuckite, Tiger's Eye. *Chakra:* past life, throat, third eye
>
>**deflect effects of:** Black Tourmaline. *Chakra:* past life, throat

cycles: Okenite. *Chakra:* past life

death, unhealed trauma: Lilac Smithsonite. *Chakra:* past life, earth, base, heart

debts, recognize: Okenite. *Chakra:* past life, solar plexus

deprivation: Prehnite. *Chakra:* past life, base, higher heart

dis-ease: Tanzanite with Iolite and Danburite. *Chakra:* past life

emotional attachments: Rainbow Aura Quartz, Rainbow Obsidian. (Wear continuously.) *Chakra:* past life

emotional pain: Charoite, Kunzite, Mangano Calcite, Tugtupite. *Chakra:* past life, heart, higher heart, solar plexus

emotional wounds: Rhodonite. *Chakra:* past life, heart, higher heart, solar plexus

entity attachment: Kunzite, Larimar, Laser Quartz, Petalite, Selenite, Smoky Amethyst. (Place on appropriate chakra, hold in place until removed, purify immediately.) *Chakra:* past life, sacral, solar plexus, third eye

family patterns: Spirit Quartz. *Chakra:* past life, sacral

grief, unhealed: Fire Opal, Spirit Quartz. *Chakra:* past life, heart

healing: Charoite, Danburite, Infinite Stone, Merlinite, Obsidian, Okenite, Pietersite, Rhodonite, Rhyolite, Voegesite. *Chakra:* past life

heart pain: Dioptase, Rhodochrosite, Rhodonite. *Chakra:* past life, higher heart

hyperactivity due to effects of: Prehnite. *Chakra:* past life, third eye

injuries: Herkimer Diamond, Onyx. *Chakra:* past life

learning from: Muscovite, Peridot. *Chakra:* past life

mental imperatives, release: Danburite, Idocrase. *Chakra:* past life

negative karma, disturbances from: Petalite

persecution: Wulfenite. *Chakra:* past life

phobias resulting from: Brandenberg Amethyst, Prehnite. *Chakra:* past life

prisoner: Idocrase. *Chakra:* past life, base

protect: Apache Tear, Jet, Labradorite, Quartz

psychosexual problems resulting from: Malachite. *Chakra:* past life, base, sacral

recall: Amber, Carnelian, Garnet, Phantom Crystals, Serpentine, Variscite. *Chakra:* past life, third eye

redress: Charoite. *Chakra:* past life

regression: Dumortierite, Green Aventurine, Variscite.

Chakra: past life, third eye

rejection: Blue Lace Agate. *Chakra:* past life, heart

relationships: Larimar, Lithium Quartz. *Chakra:* past life, base, sacral, heart

releasing vows: Banded Agate, Turquoise. *Chakra:* past life, third eye

remove blockages: Azurite, Bloodstone, Lapis Lazuli, Quartz

resentment: Rhodonite. *Chakra:* past life, base

restraint, emotional or mental: Idocrase. *Chakra:* past life, heart

sexual problems arising from: Malachite. *Chakra:* past life, base, sacral

soul agreements, recognition: Green Ridge Quartz, Wulfenite. *Chakra:* past life, higher crown

thought forms, release: Iolite. *Chakra:* past life, third eye

tie cutting: Banded Agate, Flint, Green Obsidian, Malachite, Petalite, Rainbow Mayanite, Rainbow Obsidian, Sunstone, Wulfenite. *Chakra:* past life, base, sacral, solar plexus, third eye

trauma: Ajo Blue Calcite, Blue Euclase, Cavansite, Gaia Stone, Guinea Fowl Jasper, Holly Agate, Mangano Vesuvianite, Oceanite, Oregon Opal, Peanut Wood, Ruby Lavender Quartz, Sea Sediment Jasper, Tantalite, Victorite

wound imprints in etheric body: Charoite, Flint, Novaculite, Sceptre Quartz, Selenite, Smoky Quartz,

Tibetan Black Spot Quartz wand

Peripheral circulation: Dianite, Garnet in Quartz, Ouro Verde, Riebekite with Sugilite and Bustamite. *Chakra:* dantien

Personal growth: Axinite

Personality disorders: use crystals under the guidance of a qualified crystal therapist

Personal power:

   increase: Basalt, Brandenberg Amethyst, Conichalcite, Empowerite, Eudialyte, Eye of the Storm, Orange Kyanite, Owyhee Blue Opal, Sedona Stone, Shungite, Tinguaite. *Chakra:* base, dantien

   overcome misuse of: Nuummite, Smoky Lemurian. *Chakra:* past life, base

Phobias: Andean Blue Opal, Dumortierite, Frondellite with Strengite, Girasol, Hackmanite, Oceanite. *Chakra:* past life, solar plexus, base

Physical: and see Subtle Energy Bodies page 209

   body, discomfort at being in: Candle Quartz, Empowerite, Eye of the Storm, Larvikite, Pearl Spar Dolomite, Phenacite, Picasso Jasper, Strontianite, Vanadinite (make essence by indirect method). *Chakra:* earth star, base, dantien, soma

   endurance, improve: Poppy Jasper, Schalenblende, Sodalite, Triplite. *Chakra:* earth star, base, dantien

   exhaustion: Eye of the Storm, Mariposite, Poppy Jasper, Purpurite, Strawberry Lemurian (Red Lemurian Seed Crystal), Vanadinite (make essence by

Unless otherwise directed, apply crystal over chakras, organ or site of symptom, wear as jewellery, bathe with or use as crystal essence.

indirect method). *Chakra:* earth star, base, dantien

pleasure, share: Poppy Jasper. *Chakra:* earth star, base

weakness: Diopside, Schalenblende, Sedona Stone. *Chakra:* dantien

well-being: Cloudy Quartz, Golden Healer Quartz, Guardian Stone, Keyiapo, Quantum Quattro, Que Sera, Schalenblende, Sedona Stone, Shungite. *Chakra:* earth star, base, dantien

Pineal gland: Amethyst, Apatite, Blue Moonstone, Champagne Aura Quartz, Fire and Ice Quartz, Fluorapatite, Gem Rhodonite, Moonstone, Opal, Petalite, Preseli Bluestone, Quartz, Richterite, Ruby, Sodalite, Tanzanite, Tanzine Aura Quartz, Tremolite, Yellow Labradorite. *Chakra:* third eye

Pituitary gland: Apatite, Chalcopyrite, Champagne Aura Quartz, Charoite, Elbaite, Fire and Ice Quartz, Labradorite, Rhodonite, Sugilite Tanzine Aura Quartz. *Chakra:* third eye

Pomposity: Turritella Agate

'Poor me' syndrome: Lemurian Jade

Post Traumatic Stress disorder: Bird's Eye Jasper, Eisenkiesel, Empowerite, Eye of the Storm, Richterite, Shungite, Tantalite, Victorite. *Chakra:* dantien, higher heart

Poverty consciousness: Citrine Herkimer, Smoky Citrine, Tugtupite. *Chakra:* sacral

Powerlessness: Basalt, Eye of the Storm, Nuummite, Smoky Elestial Quartz. *Chakra:* base, dantien

---

Unless otherwise directed, apply crystal over chakras, organ or site of symptom, wear as jewellery, bathe with or use as crystal essence.

Prostate: Brochantite, Bustamite, Schalenblende. *Chakra:* base

   enlarged: Calcite Fairy Stone

Psychological:

   autonomy: Pyrophyllite, Xenotine. *Chakra:* dantien

   balance: Amblygonite

   catharsis: Barite, Epidote, Gaia Stone, Nirvana Quartz, Smoky Elestial Quartz, Smoky Spirit Quartz

   healing: Agrellite, Ajoite, Annabergite, Black Kyanite, Diopside, Flint, Fulgarite, Lemurian Jade, Lemurian Seed, Nuummite, Ocean Jasper, Quantum Quattro, Smoky Elestial, Stellar Beam Calcite

   insights: Actinolite, Lazulite, Leopardskin Serpentine, Septarian, Shiva Lingham, Smoky Brandenberg Amethyst

   safety: Tree Agate, Xenotine

   shadow: Agrellite, Azeztulite with Morganite, Champagne Aura Quartz, Covellite, Day and Night Quartz, Lazulite, Lemurian Seed, Molybdenite, Nuummite, Phantom Quartz, Proustite, Shaman Quartz, Smoky Elestial Quartz, Voegesite. *Chakra:* solar plexus

   union: Graphic Smoky Quartz, Zebra Stone, Zircon

Psychosexual problems: Eilat Stone. *Chakra:* base, sacral

Psychosomatic disease: Andescine Labradorite, Angel's Wing Calcite, Astraline, Azeztulite with Morganite, Azotic Topaz, Benitoite, Dumortierite, Fire Obsidian, Gaia Stone, Golden Danburite, Icicle Calcite, Larvikite,

Ocean Blue Jasper, Roselite, Snakeskin Pyrite, Titanite (Sphene), Voegesite. *Chakra:* third eye, higher heart

sexual: Azeztulite with Morganite

stabilize body during changes: Basalt, Huebnerite, Luxullianite, Nunderite, Snakeskin Pyrite, Tangerose

understand causes of: Azotic Topaz, Benitoite, Chalcopyrite, Faden Quartz, Icicle Calcite, Kornerupine, Stichtite and Serpentine, Voegesite

Pulse, irregular: Agate, Charoite. Wear over heart.

– Q –

Qi: Aquamarine, Carnelian, Eye of the Storm, Garnet, Poppy Jasper, Quantum Quattro, Red Amethyst, Red Jasper, Red Zincite, Ruby, Triplite. *Chakra:* higher heart, base or dantien. Wear continuously.

depleted: Ammolite, Budd Stone (African Jade), Chalcopyrite, Eye of the Storm (Judy's Jasper), Granite, Kyanite, Magnetite (Lodestone), Poppy Jasper, Que Sera, Red Amethyst, Rhodozite, Ruby in Granite, Sonora Sunrise, Violane, Witches Finger, Zincite. *Chakra:* sacral, dantien

transmit: Feather Pyrite, Green Ridge Quartz, Que Sera, Rhodozite, Terraluminite

– R –

Raynaud's disease: Blue or White Aragonite, Dianite, Ouro Verde, Reinerite. *Chakra:* dantien

Relaxation: Amethyst, Aventurine, Blue Calcite, Dioptase, Fire Agate, Fuchsite, Golden Calcite, Jasper, Magnesite, Peridot, Rhodonite, Smoky Quartz

Release anger and tension: Alabaster, Blue Phantom Quartz, Chinese Red Quartz, Cinnabar in Jasper, Ethiopian Opal, Greenlandite, Nzuri Moyo, Pearl Spar Dolomite, Phosphosiderite, Tugtupite, Ussingite. *Chakra:* base, dantien

Repair, assist body to: Aegirine, Bixbite, Brandenberg Amethyst, Celestial Quartz, Molybdenite, Quantum Quattro Rutile with Hematite, Rutilated Quartz, Shungite, Zoisite. *Chakra:* dantien

Repressed:

    anger: Cinnabar in Jasper, Ethiopian Opal, Nzuri Moyo, Phosphosiderite. *Chakra:* base, dantien

    emotions: Ethiopian Opal

Reproductive system: Beryllonite, Black Kyanite, Calcite Fairy Stone, Fire and Ice Quartz, Lepidocrosite, Menalite, Voegesite, Xenotine. *Chakra:* base, sacral, dantien

    fallopian tubes: Menalite, Schalenblende. *Chakra:* sacral

    female: Black Moonstone, Fire and Ice Quartz, Menalite, Schalenblende, Tangerose. *Chakra:* sacral, base

inflammation: Blue Euclase, Dendritic Chalcedony, Hanksite, Kundalini Quartz, Rhodozite, Sulphur in Quartz

male: Calcite Fairy Stone, Schalenblende, Shiva Lingam

ovaries: Menalite, Schalenblende

testicles: Alexandrite, Schalenblende. *Chakra:* base

Resistance to change: Dragon Stone, Eclipse Stone, Luxullianite, Montebrasite, Snakeskin Pyrite, Tangerose. *Chakra:* base, dantien, heart

Respiratory system: Blue Aragonite, Cacoxenite, Halite, Kambaba Jasper, Merlinite, Prophecy Stone, Pyrite in Quartz, Quantum Quattro, Richterite, Riebekite with Sugilite and Bustamite, Smoky Amethyst, Snakeskin Pyrite, Stromatolite, Tremolite. *Chakra:* dantien, higher heart

problems: Cacoxenite, Kambaba Jasper, Riebekite with Sugilite and Bustamite, Smoky Amethyst, Stromatolite, Tremolite

Retrieval, child or soul parts: Fulgarite, Khutnohorite, Tangerose

RNA stabilizing: Chalcopyrite. *Chakra:* dantien

– S –

Saviour complex: Cassiterite

Scapegoating behaviour: Champagne Aura Quartz, Mohawkite, Scapolite, Smoky Amethyst

Seasonal affective disorder: Sunshine Aura Quartz, Sunstone, Topaz, Triplite. Wear continuously.

Security issues: Chinese Red Quartz, Nzuri Moyo. *Chakra:* base

    emotional: Mangano Vesuvianite, Oceanite, Tugtupite. *Chakra:* base, dantien, solar plexus

    letting go of: Axinite, Scheelite. *Chakra:* base, dantien

Self:

    acceptance: Lavender Quartz, Lemurian Seed, Orange Phantom, Peach Selenite, Quantum Quattro, Tangerose, Tugtupite. *Chakra:* heart, higher heart

    awareness: Citrine Spirit Quartz

    confidence: Blue Quartz, Lemurian Seed, Nunderite, Pink Sunstone

    criticism: Epidote

    deception: Oregon Opal

    defeating programs: Desert Rose, Drusy Quartz, Kinoite, Nuummite, Paraiba Tourmaline, Quantum Quattro, Strawberry Quartz

    development: Hemimorphite

    discipline: Blue Quartz, Dumortierite, Scapolite, Sillimanite

    doubt: Rosophia

Unless otherwise directed, apply crystal over chakras, organ or site of symptom, wear as jewellery, bathe with or use as crystal essence.

esteem: Eisenkiesel, Graphic Smoky Quartz (Zebra Stone), Hackmanite, Lazulite, Morion, Nzuri Moyo, Pink Phantom, Strawberry Quartz, Tinguaite. *Chakra:* base, sacral, dantien, heart, higher heart

expression: Eilat Stone, Mariposite, Owyhee Blue Opal. *Chakra:* throat

forgiveness: Chinese Red Quartz, Eudialyte, Pink Crackle Quartz, Spirit Quartz, Steatite, Tugtupite

hatred (combating): Blizzard Stone, Quantum Quattro, Tugtupite. *Chakra:* base

healing: Benitoite, Elestial Quartz, Eudialyte, Faden Quartz, Gaia Stone, Morion, Quantum Quattro, Rosophia, Septarian

image, poor: Dianite, Kinoite, Trummer Jasper

integrating: Ajoite, Amethyst Herkimer, Brandenberg, Eilat Stone, Faden Quartz, Quantum Quattro, Sichuan Quartz

nurturing: Poppy Jasper, Quantum Quattro, Septarian, Smoky Cathedral Quartz, Super 7

pity: Epidote

preservation: Dumortierite

respect: Rainforest Jasper

sabotaging behaviour: Agrellite, Quantum Quattro, Scapolite

sufficiency: Nunderite, Quantum Quattro. *Chakra:* base

trust: Honey Calcite. *Chakra:* sacral

worth: Rose Aura Quartz. *Chakra:* base, sacral

Unless otherwise directed, apply crystal over chakras, organ or site of symptom, wear as jewellery, bathe with or use as crystal essence.

Senile dementia: Anthrophyllite, Chalcedony, Rose Quartz, Stichtite and Serpentine. *Chakra:* third eye. Base of skull or wear continuously.

Senior moments: Barite, Blue or Black Moonstone, Hematoid Calcite, Herderite, Marcasite, Vivianite. *Chakra:* third eye. Or place at base of skull.

Sensory organs, desensitized: Schalenblende. *Chakra:* dantien

Sexual:

> **abuse, healing:** Apricot Quartz, Azeztulite with Morganite, Eilat Stone, Honey Opal, Lazurine, Orange Kyanite, Pink Crackle Quartz, Proustite, Shiva Lingam, Xenotine. *Chakra:* base, sacral, dantien
>
> **dysfunction:** Orange Kyanite
>
> **libido, loss of:** Orange Kyanite, Poppy Jasper, Shiva Lingam, Shungite. *Chakra:* base, sacral, dantien
>
> **organs:** Menalite, Shiva Lingam. *Chakra:* base, sacral
>
> **pleasure, prolong:** Poppy Jasper. *Chakra:* base, sacral

Shadow, integrate: Morion, Proustite, Smoky Lemurian Seed, Voegesite

Shamanic anchor: see Anchor page 216

Shamanic journey: Brandenberg Amethyst, Celestobarite, Chrysotile in Serpentine, Graphic Smoky Quartz (Zebra Stone), Leopardskin Jasper, Lodolite, Mount Shasta Opal, Nunderite, Owyhee Blue Opal, Polychrome Jasper, Scolecite, Serpentine in Obsidian, Shaman Quartz, Smoky Quartz with Aegirine, Stibnite, Titanite (Sphene). See also Journeying page 275.

Unless otherwise directed, apply crystal over chakras, organ or site of symptom, wear as jewellery, bathe with or use as crystal essence.

Shame: Azeztulite with Morganite, Catlinite. *Chakra:* base, dantien

Shape shifting: Leopardskin Jasper, Mount Shasta Opal, Serpentine in Obsidian. *Chakra:* soma/third eye

Shield yourself: Black Tourmaline, Healer's Gold, Mohawkite, Nuummite, Polychrome Jasper, Pyrite, Shieldite, Shungite, Smoky Quartz, Tantalite. *Chakra:* higher heart

Shock: Eye of the Storm (Judy's Jasper), Quantum Quattro, Que Sera, Richterite, Smoky Elestial Quartz, Tantalite. *Chakra:* solar plexus (take crystal essence frequently or wear stones constantly)

    anaphylactic: Ouro Verde

Shoulders: Empowerite, Prehnite with Epidote, Scapolite

    frozen: Ice Quartz. *Chakra:* throat

    psychosomatic reasons behind frozen: Gaia Stone, Prehnite with Epidote, Scapolite

Skeletal system: Coprolite, Crinoidal Limestone, Empowerite, Golden Coracalcite, Limonite, Pearl Spar Dolomite, Phantom Calcite, Poldervaarite, Pyromorphite, Steatite, Stromatolite, Tinguaite, Turritella Agate. *Chakra:* third eye

    flexibility, improve: Coprolite, Kimberlite, Tinguaite

    support growth in youth: Limonite

Sleep: see Insomnia page 270

Sluggishness: Poppy Jasper, Quantum Quattro, Que Sera. *Chakra:* base, dantien

Smell, restore sense of: Fluorapatite

Unless otherwise directed, apply crystal over chakras, organ or site of symptom, wear as jewellery, bathe with or use as crystal essence.

Soul: Brandenberg Amethyst, Cathedral Quartz, Golden Danburite, Nirvana Quartz, Trigonic Quartz. *Chakra:* higher crown, heart

> **cleanser:** Anandalite, Black Kyanite, Brandenberg Amethyst, Chinese Chromium Quartz, Chrysotile in Serpentine, Golden Danburite, Khutnohorite, Prehnite with Epidote, Rutile with Hematite, Smoky Cathedral Quartz, Smoky Elestial Quartz

> **contracts, release:** Black Kyanite, Boli Stone, Brandenberg Amethyst, Dumortierite, Gabbro, Kakortokite, Leopardskin Jasper, Pyrophyllite, Red Amethyst, Wind Fossil Agate

> **dark night of:** Golden Danburite, Khutnohorite, Stone of Sanctuary

> **encrustations:** Ethiopian Opal

> **evolution:** Hilulite, Paraiba Tourmaline, Shift Crystal

> **growth:** Agrellite, Beryllonite, Epidote

> **healing:** Amphibole, Black Kyanite, Blue Aragonite, Brandenberg Amethyst, Cassiterite, Ethiopian Opal, Fiskenaesset Ruby, Khutnohorite, Marble, Nuummite, Pink Lazurine, Porphyrite (Chinese Letter Stone), Preseli Bluestone, Ruby Lavender Quartz, Trigonic Quartz

> **imperatives:** Nirvana Quartz, Porphyrite (Chinese Letter Stone), Tantalite

> **incarnate fully:** Bushman Red Cascade Quartz, Celestial Quartz, Snakeskin Agate

> **memory:** Amphibole, Cacoxenite, Datolite, Trigonic

Quartz

overcome fear in: Amphibole, Khutnohorite, Revelation Stone, Stone of Sanctuary, Tangerose

overlay: Scheelite

path/plan: Amblygonite, Anthrophyllite, Astrophyllite, Black Kyanite, Blue Aragonite, Brazilianite, Candle Quartz, Cathedral Quartz, Crystalline Kyanite, Datolite, Golden Danburite, Icicle Calcite, Indicolite Quartz, Khutnohorite, Lemurian Jade, Leopardskin Serpentine, Lepidocrosite, Merkabite Calcite, Paraiba Tourmaline, Rainbow Mayanite, Rainbow Moonstone, Stellar Beam Calcite

retrieval: Epidote, Faden Quartz, Fulgarite, Gaspeite, Khutnohorite, Mount Shasta Opal, Nuummite, Preseli Bluestone, Rainbow Mayanite, Snakeskin Agate, Tangerose. *Chakra:* higher heart, third eye

Spasms: Amazonite, Aragonite, Azurite, Carnelian, Electric-blue Obsidian, Magnesite, Ruby

Spinal:

alignment: Blue Moonstone, Graphic Smoky Quartz (Zebra Stone), Huebnerite, Phantom Selenite, Scolecite, Shell Jasper, Stichtite, Tinguaite

column: Calcite Fairy Stone, Huebnerite, Scolecite, Tinguaite

energy, blocked: Flame Aura Quartz, Garnet in Quartz, Sedona Stone, Strawberry Lemurian

inflexible: Blue Moonstone, Phantom Selenite, Scolecite, Tinguaite

Unless otherwise directed, apply crystal over chakras, organ or site of symptom, wear as jewellery, bathe with or use as crystal essence.

injuries: Cathedral Quartz

out of alignment: Blue Moonstone, Graphic Smoky Quartz (Zebra Stone), Rainbow Moonstone, Scolecite, Tinguaite, Vivianite

strengthen: Erythrite

Spirit release: Nirvana Quartz and see entity attachment page 302

Spiritual:

development: Agnitite, Ajo Quartz, Anandalite, Andara Glass, Andescine Labradorite, Angel's Wing Calcite, Auralite 23, Azeztulite, Carrolite, Celestobarite, Dianite, Eclipse Stone, Epiphany Quartz, Fire and Ice, Fire Obsidian, Firework Obsidian, Galaxyite, Glaucophane, Glendonite, Golden Coracalcite, Golden Healer, Green Ridge Quartz, Kambaba Jasper, Larvikite, Lodolite, Petrified Wood, Phlogopite, Prehnite with Epidote, Que Sera, Rainbow Mayanite, Ruby Lavender Quartz, Sedona Stone, Shell Jasper, Tantalite, Terraluminite, Titanite (Sphene), Violane

blocked: Andara Glass, Auralite 23, Bumble Bee Jasper, Celestobarite, Master Shamanite, Realgar, Rutilated Kunzite, Sedona Stone, Terraluminite, Titanite, Victorite

interference: Mohawkite, Nunderite, Polychrome Jasper, Rainbow Mayanite, Tantalite. *Chakra:* crown (wear constantly)

Spleen: Aegirine, Amber, Apple Aura Quartz,

Aquamarine, Aventurine, Azurite, Black Moonstone, Bloodstone, Blue Quartz, Brochantite, Bustamite, Chalcedony, Cinnabar in Jasper, Citrine, Fluorite, Gaspeite, Green Obsidian, Guinea Fowl Jasper, Jade, Marcasite, Mookaite Jasper, Nunderite, Orange River Quartz, Peridot, Red Obsidian, Red Tourmaline, Ruby, Septarian, Sunstone, Yellow Labradorite, Wulfenite, Zircon. *Chakra:* spleen

   blood flow: Mookaite Jasper

   detoxifying: Amechlorite, Banded Agate, Chlorite Quartz, Eye of the Storm, Jamesonite, Larvikite, Pyrite in Magnesite, Rainbow Covellite, Richterite, Seraphinite, Shungite, Smoky Quartz with Aegirine

   protection: Aventurine, Gaspeite, Green Aventurine, Jade, Nunderite, Tugtupite

Stability: Celestobarite, Eye of the Storm, Smoky Elestial Quartz. *Chakra:* base, dantien

Stagnant energy: Black Tourmaline, Calcite, Chrome Diopside, Clear Topaz, Eye of the Storm, Garnet in Quartz, Orgonite, Poppy Jasper, Ruby Lavender Quartz, Sedona Stone, Shaman Quartz, Shungite, Smoky Quartz, Spirit Quartz, Tantalite and see negative energy page 294. *Chakra:* base, dantien

Stamina: Anthrophyllite, Epidote, Purpurite. *Chakra:* base, dantien

Stammering: Greenlandite. *Chakra:* throat, third eye

Star being, contact: Aswan Granite, Glaucophane, Lemurian Seed, Mount Shasta Opal, Scolecite, Star

Hollandite, Starseed Quartz, Sugar Blade Quartz

Star children: Calcite Fairy Stone, Empowerite, Fairy Quartz, Glaucophane, Star Hollandite, Starseed Quartz. *Chakra:* higher crown

Stomach: Amblygonite, Bismuth, Black Moonstone, Bytownite, Cryolite, Mookaite Jasper, Paraiba Tourmaline, Prasiolite, Serpentine in Obsidian, Snakeskin Agate, Stibnite, Turritella Agate, Tugtupite. *Chakra:* solar plexus

Strengthen chakras: Magnetite (Lodestone), Quartz and see Chakras page 209

Stress: Amber, Amethyst, Andean Blue Opal, Aquamarine, Atlantasite, Aventurine, Basalt, Beryl, Bird's Eye Jasper, Brandenberg Amethyst, Bronzite, Cacoxenite, Charoite, Dioptase, Dumortierite, Eisenkiesel, Eye of the Storm, Gabbro, Galaxyite, Golden Healer Quartz, Graphic Smoky Quartz, Green Aventurine, Green Diopside, Hematoid Calcite, Herkimer Diamond, Jade, Jasper, Labradorite, Lapis Lazuli, Magnetite, Marble, Mariposite, Mount Shasta Opal, Nuummite, Ocean Jasper, Paraiba Tourmaline, Petalite, Pyrite in Magnesite, Quantum Quattro, Que Sera, Red Amethyst, Rhodonite, Richterite, Riebekite with Sugilite and Bustamite, Rose Quartz, Serpentine, Shungite, Siberian Quartz, Smoky Quartz, Sodalite, Vera Cruz Amethyst

> **related illness:** Ajoite with Shattuckite, Amechlorite, Blue Aragonite, Blue Siberian Quartz, Bustamite, Candle Quartz, Epidote, Fiskenaesset Ruby, Morion,

Mount Shasta Opal, Quantum Quattro, Riebekite with Sugilite and Bustamite. *Chakra:* third eye, heart, solar plexus

Superiority: Heulandite. *Chakra:* dantien

Supra-adrenals: Amber, Amethyst, Aquamarine, Axinite, Beryl, Cacoxenite, Charoite, Dioptase, Epidote, Eye of the Storm, Gaspeite, Green Aventurine, Herkimer Diamond, Jasper, Labradorite, Lapis Lazuli, Magnetite (Lodestone), Nunderite, Petalite, Picrolite, Rhodonite, Richterite, Rose Quartz, Siberian Quartz. *Chakra:* dantien. Or tape over kidneys.

Subtle energy bodies: see Energy bodies page 209

Sympathetic nervous system: Cumberlandite, Golden Healer Quartz

– T –

Tachycardia: Amber, Ammolite, Danburite, Garnet, Purpurite, Rose Quartz, Tugtupite. *Chakra:* dantien, heart

Taking on other people's feelings or conditions: Brochantite, Healer's Gold, Iridescent Pyrite, Lemurian Jade, Mohawkite. *Chakra:* solar plexus, spleen

Tantric practices: Anandalite™, Eudialyte, Kundalini Quartz, Serpentine in Obsidian, Tiffany Stone, Victorite

Taste, loss of: Mystic Topaz

T-cells: Bloodstone, Diaspore (Zultanite), Dioptase, Klinoptilolith, Quantum Quattro, Que Sera, Richterite, Rosophia, Shungite, Tangerine Sun Aura Quartz, Tangerose and see Immune system page 269. *Chakra:* higher heart

Teeth: Brookite, Cavansite, Fluorapatite, Glendonite, Molybdenite, Paraiba Tourmaline, Phlogopite, Poldervaarite, Pyrite in Magnesite, Shell Jasper, Stichtite, Stromatolite, Strontianite, Titanite (Sphene), Winchite, Wind Fossil Agate

Telepathy: Afghanite, Arsenopyrite, Auralite 23, Avalonite, Blue Selenite, Blue Siberian Quartz, Eilat Stone, Limonite, Red Amethyst, Sichuan Quartz, Tanzanite

Temperature, regulate: Crackled Fire Agate, Dinosaur Bone, Nuummite, Pyrite in Magnesite (place beside left ear)

Unless otherwise directed, apply crystal over chakras, organ or site of symptom, wear as jewellery, bathe with or use as crystal essence.

Temper tantrums: Neptunite, Pearl Spar Dolomite. *Chakra:* base, dantien

Thought form, disperse: Aegirine, Firework Obsidian, Nuummite, Rainbow Mayanite, Scolecite, Smoky Amethyst, Smoky Citrine, Spectrolite, Stibnite

Thoughts racing: Auralite 23, Blue Selenite, Pearl Spar Dolomite, Rhomboid Calcite, Scolecite

Three-chambered heart chakra, open: Lemurian Aquitane Calcite, Mangano Calcite, Petalite, Rosophia, Tugtupite and see Heart, Heart Seed and Higher Heart chakras pages 199–201

Throat: Blue Quartz, Blue Siberian Quartz, Chrysotile, Chrysotile in Serpentine, Eclipse Stone, Glaucophane, Indicolite Quartz, Owyhee Blue Opal, Paraiba Tourmaline, Stromatolite. *Chakra:* throat

   encourage production: Diaspore, Golden Healer Quartz, Klinoptilolith, Quantum Quattro, Que Sera, Shungite, Tangerose

Thymus: Amethyst, Andean Opal, Angelite, Aqua Aura, Aventurine, Bloodstone, Blue or Green Tourmaline, Blue Halite, Chrysotile, Citrine, Diaspore, Dioptase, Eilat Stone, Hiddenite, Indicolite Quartz, Jadeite, Klinoptilolith, Lapis Lazuli, Peridot, Prehnite with Epidote, Quantum Quattro, Quartz, Que Sera, Richterite, Rose Quartz, Septarian, Shaman Quartz, Stromatolite, Thompsonite, Tremolite. *Chakra:* higher heart

   underactive: Aqua Aura Quartz, Eilat Stone, Hiddenite, Lapis Lazuli, Peridot, Quantum Quattro,

Que Sera, Smithsonite

Thyroid: Amber, Aqua Aura, Aquamarine, Azurite, Beryl, Blue Halite, Blue Tourmaline, Candle Quartz, Celestite, Champagne Aura Quartz, Citrine, Cryolite, Cumberlandite, Eilat Stone, Idocrase, Indicolite Quartz, Kyanite, Lapis Lazuli, Lavender Aura Quartz, Lazulite, Leopardskin Serpentine, Paraiba Tourmaline, Prehnite with Epidote, Quantum Quattro, Rhodonite, Richterite, Rutilated Quartz, Sapphire, Sodalite, Turquoise, Vanadinite (make essence by indirect method). *Chakra:* throat

> **balance:** Aquamarine, Cacoxenite, Richterite
>
> **deficiencies:** Angelite, Blue Lace Agate, Citrine, Harlequin Quartz, Kyanite, Lapis Lazuli, Tanzine Aura Quartz
>
> **regulate:** Lapis Lazuli, Rhodonite, Richterite, Tanzine Aura Quartz
>
> **stimulate:** Rhodonite, Rutilated Quartz, Tanzine Aura Quartz. *Chakra:* throat

Tiredness, chronic: Amethyst, Bismuth, Carnelian, Chlorite Quartz, Cinnabar Jasper, Eudialyte, Eye of the Storm, Fire Agate, Fire Obsidian, Golden Healer Quartz, Hematite, Iron Pyrite, Poppy Jasper, Purpurite, Quantum Quattro, Que Sera, Red Jasper, Rose Quartz, Ruby, Ruby in Fuchsite, Tiger Iron, Triplite, and see Fatigue page 259. *Chakra*: base, dantien

Tissue:

> **connective:** Desert Rose, Greenlandite, Piemontite,

Prehnite with Epidote

degeneration: Alexandrite, Eilat Stone, Tantalite

detoxify: Amechlorite, Eye of the Storm, Fairy Quartz, Jamesonite, Larvikite, Phlogopite, Pyrite in Magnesite, Rainbow Covellite, Richterite, Shungite, Smoky Amethyst, Smoky Quartz with Aegirine, Tantalite

hardened: Prehnite with Epidote, Pumice

regeneration: Alexandrite, Eilat Stone, Flint, Leopardskin Jasper, Nuummite, Tantalite

repair: Alexandrite, Diaspore (Zultanite), Eilat Stone, Eisenkiesel, Flint, Greenlandite, Khutnohorite, Piemontite, Rutilated Quartz, Tantalite

Toxicity: Amber, Arsenopyrite, Champagne Aura Quartz, Chlorite Quartz, Green Jasper, Klinoptilolith, Morion Quartz, Orgonite, Rutilated Quartz, Shieldite, Smoky Elestial Quartz, Smoky Quartz, Snakeskin Pyrite, Sodalite, Sunshine Aura Quartz, Tourmalinated Quartz, Valentinite and Stibnite. *Chakra:* dantien, earth, spleen. Place in environment.

Toxins: see Detoxification page 245. *Chakra:* earth star, spleen

disperse: Actinolite, Aegirine, Ametrine, Banded Agate, Barite, Blue Quartz, Celestite, Celestobarite, Champagne Aura Quartz, Chinese Chlorite Quartz, Chromium Quartz, Chrysanthemum Stone, Conichalcite, Covellite, Danburite with Chlorite, Eilat Stone, Epidote, Eye of the Storm, Fairy Quartz,

Fiskenaesset Ruby, Golden Danburite, Halite, Hanksite, Huebnerite, Iolite, Leopardskin Serpentine, Morion, Ocean Jasper, Orgonite, Pearl Spar Dolomite, Poppy Jasper, Pumice, Pyrite in Quartz, Quantum Quattro, Seraphinite, Serpentine, Shieldite, Smoky Elestial Quartz, Smoky Herkimer, Snakeskin Pyrite, Sodalite, Spirit Quartz, Yellow Apatite. *Chakra:* base, earth star, dantien, spleen, solar plexus

disperse from environment: Chlorite Quartz, Chrysanthemum Stone, Orgonite, Shieldite, Shungite, Sodalite

remove: Ametrine, Celestite, Chlorite Quartz, Iolite, Moss Agate, Orgonite, Serpentine, Shieldite, Shungite, Sodalite, Yellow Apatite. *Chakra:* base, earth, spleen, solar plexus

strengthen resistance to: Beryl, Eye of the Storm, Klinoptilolith, Ocean Jasper, Pyrite in Quartz, Shungite. *Chakra:* base, earth star, dantien, spleen, solar plexus

Tranquillizer: Amblygonite, Blue Quartz, Candle Quartz, Eye of the Storm, Leopardskin Jasper, Poppy Jasper, Pounamu Jade, Quantum Quattro, Strawberry Quartz, Vera Cruz Amethyst. *Chakra:* higher heart

Trauma: Ammolite, Blue Euclase, Bornite, Brandenberg Amethyst, Cathedral Quartz, Cavansite, Dumortierite, Empowerite, Epidote, Faden Quartz, Fulgarite, Gaia Stone, Garnet in Quartz, Goethite, Green Diopside, Green Ridge Quartz, Guardian Stone, Kimberlite, Mangano

Vesuvianite, Novaculite with Nuummite, Ocean Blue Jasper, Oregon Opal, Peach Selenite, Peanut Wood, Prasiolite, Richterite, Ruby Lavender Quartz, Scapolite, Sea Sediment Jasper, Smoky Elestial, Spirit Quartz, Tantalite, Victorite, Wavellite, Youngite. *Chakra:* solar plexus (or wear constantly)

Triple burner meridian, rebalance: Crackled Fire Agate, Nuummite (place in front of left ear)

Twitching/tics: Blue Euclase, Bronzite, Cat's Eye Quartz, Dumortierite, Orange Moss Agate, Pyrite in Magnesite, Serpentine in Obsidian, Smoky Amethyst

– U –

Unconditional self-love: Citrine, Emerald, Mangano Calcite, Pink Calcite, Rose Quartz, Tugtupite

Ungroundedness: Aztee, Basalt, Celestobarite, Chlorite Quartz, Dragon Stone, Empowerite, Flint, Granite, Graphic Smoky Quartz (Zebra Stone), Hematite, Kambaba Jasper, Mohawkite, Peanut Wood, Polychrome Jasper, Proustite, Serpentine in Obsidian, Shell Jasper, Smoky Elestial Quartz, Steatite, Stromatolite. *Chakra:* earth star, base, dantien, Gaia. Or place behind knees.

Unite:

> **and activate all chakras and energy bodies:** Anandalite, Brandenberg Amethyst, Green Ridge Quartz, Phenacite
>
> **base and crown:** Harlequin Quartz, Red Amethyst
>
> **earth star to soul star and stellar gateway:** Celestobarite, or Blue Kyanite with Preseli Bluestone on base of skull and Flint on earth star
>
> **third eye, soma, alta major, crown, stellar gateway and soul star:** Afghanite

– V –

Vampirism of heart energy: Gaspeite, Greenlandite, Iridescent Pyrite, Lemurian Aquitane Calcite, Nunderite, Tantalite, Xenotine. *Chakra:* solar plexus, heart, higher

---

Unless otherwise directed, apply crystal over chakras, organ or site of symptom, wear as jewellery, bathe with or use as crystal essence.

heart

Vampirism of spleen energy: Gaspeite, Iridescent Pyrite, Nunderite, Tantalite, Xenotine. *Chakra:* spleen

Vertigo: Celestobarite, Dogtooth Calcite, Fairy Quartz, Zircon (place on back of neck)

Vibrational change, facilitate: Anandalite, Bismuth, Gabbro, Huebnerite, Lemurian Gold Opal, Lemurian Jade, Lemurian Seed, Luxullianite, Montebrasite, Mtrolite, Nunderite, Rainbow Mayanite, Rosophia, Sanda Rosa Azeztulite, Snakeskin Pyrite, Sonora Sunrise, Trigonic Quartz. *Chakra:* higher heart, higher crown (wear stones frequently or keep within reach and hold frequently)

Victim mentality: Amblygonite, Brazilianite, Epidote, Green Ridge Quartz, Hematoid Calcite, Ice Quartz, Marcasite, Orange River Quartz, Smoky Lemurian Seed, Tugtupite with Nuummite, Zircon. *Chakra:* dantien

– W –

Weak:

    energy field: Celestobarite, Chlorite Quartz, Chrome Diopside, Orgonite, Poppy Jasper, Quantum Quattro, Que Sera, Sedona Stone. Hold between sacral and solar plexus.

Weather sensitivity: Apricot Quartz, Avalonite, Chlorite Quartz, Golden Healer Quartz, Golden Pietersite,

Khutnohorite, Quantum Quattro, Que Sera, Pietersite, Poppy Jasper, Shell Jasper, Shungite, Sillimanite, Silver Leaf Jasper, Trummer Jasper, Wonder Stone. *Chakra:* third eye

Well-being, promote: Beryllonite, Fiskenaesset Ruby, Fulgarite, Ice Quartz, Keyiapo, Quantum Quattro, Que Sera, Shift Crystal, Strawberry Quartz, Tugtupite, Ussingite. *Chakra:* higher heart

Worry, excessive: Pink Crackle Quartz, Revelation Stone, Snakeskin Agate, Sonora Sunrise

– X –

Xiphoid process: see Heart Seed chakra page 200

– Y –

Yin-yang balance: Alunite, Amphibole, Black Onyx, Celestite, Citrine, Dalmatian Stone, Day and Night Quartz, Eilat Stone, Hematite, Hematite with Rutile, Kyanite, Merlinite, Morion, Onyx, Poppy Jasper, Scheelite, Shiva Lingam, Spirit Quartz. *Chakra:* base, sacral, dantien or wear continuously

---

Unless otherwise directed, apply crystal over chakras, organ or site of symptom, wear as jewellery, bathe with or use as crystal essence.

– Z –

Zest for life: Bushman Red Cascade Quartz, Carnelian, Orange River Quartz, Poppy Jasper, Red Jasper, Zebra Stone. *Chakra:* dantien

Unless otherwise directed, apply crystal over chakras, organ or site of symptom, wear as jewellery, bathe with or use as crystal essence.

Footnotes

1. "Detection of extraordinary large bio-magnetic field strength from human hand during external Qi emission." Seto, A; Kusaka, C; Nakazato, S; Huang, WR; Sato, T; Hisamitsu, T; Takeshige, C. *Acupunct Electrother Res.* 1992;17(2):75–94.
2. Many of the descriptions and definitions are shared across numerous sites without attribution so apologies if you were the original source and it isn't acknowledged here.
3. The same text is found in *Walking In The Light* by Peter Fust and on many websites.

Resources

Crystals

Crystals specially attuned for you by Judy Hall are available from: www.angeladditions.co.uk

Trigonics, Eye of the Storm and just about everything else can be obtained from: www.exquisitecrystals.com

Essences

Petaltone cleansing and recharging essences: www.petaltone.co.uk

Crystal Balance cleansing and recharging essences: www.crystalbalance.net

Green Man essences: www.greenmanshop.co.uk

Further reading

Hall, Judy:

Crystal Prescriptions volumes 1–3 (O-Books)

The Encyclopedia of Crystals (Hamlyn/Fair Winds Press)

Earth Blessings: Using Crystals for Personal Energy Clearing, Earth Healing and Environmental Enhancement (Watkins Publishing)

Judy Hall's Book of Psychic Development (Flying Horse)

Good Vibrations (Flying Horse)

Crystal Bible volumes 1–3 (Godsfield Press)

The Crystal Wisdom Oracle (Watkins Publishing)

Crystals and Sacred Sites (Fair Winds Press/Quarto)

Crystals (Hay House Basics)
101 Power Crystals (Fair Winds Press/Quarto)
Crystal Healing Pack (Godsfield Press)

Lilly, Sue and Simon:
Crystal, Colour and Chakra Healing: How to Harness the Transforming Powers of Colour, Crystals and Your Body's Own Subtle Energies to Increase Health and Well Being

Research and relevant reports

Scientific Study of Kundalini Activation and Its Benefits
http://www.nithyananda.org/article/scientific-study-kundalini-activation-its-benefits#gsc.tab=0

The Kundalini Database Project https://www.emerging-sciences.org/kdp/?gclid=CMehzdWWisMCFTLJtAody1UALA

Why Study Kundalini?
http://www.icrcanada.org/research/approach/whystudykundalini

On A Possible Psychophysiology of the Yogic Chakra System, SM Roney-Dougal, PhD
http://www.psi-researchcentre.co.uk/article_2.html

Coming to Grips with the Divine
https://bodydivineyoga.wordpress.com/tag/hand-chakra

The Crystal Palace
http://biologyofkundalini.com/article.php?story=TheCry
stalPalace&query=crystal%2Bpalace

Crystal healing training

In the UK:
The Institute of Crystal and Gem Therapists
http://www.icgt.co.uk

BOOKS

SPIRITUALITY

O is a symbol of the world, of oneness and unity; this eye represents knowledge and insight. We publish titles on general spirituality and living a spiritual life. We aim to inform and help you on your own journey in this life.
If you have enjoyed this book, why not tell other readers by posting a review on your preferred book site?

Recent bestsellers from O-Books are:

Heart of Tantric Sex
Diana Richardson
Revealing Eastern secrets of deep love and intimacy to
Western couples.
Paperback: 978-1-90381-637-0 ebook: 978-1-84694-637-0

Crystal Prescriptions
The A-Z guide to over 1,200 symptoms and their healing
crystals
Judy Hall
The first in the popular series of seven books, this
handy little guide is packed as tight as a pill-bottle with
crystal remedies for ailments.
Paperback: 978-1-90504-740-6 ebook: 978-1-84694-629-5

Take Me To Truth
Undoing the Ego
Nouk Sanchez, Tomas Vieira
The best-selling step-by-step book on shedding the Ego,
using the teachings of *A Course In Miracles*.
Paperback: 978-1-84694-050-7 ebook: 978-1-84694-654-7

The 7 Myths about Love...Actually!
The journey from your HEAD to the HEART of your SOUL
Mike George
Smashes all the myths about LOVE.
Paperback: 978-1-84694-288-4 ebook: 978-1-84694-682-0

The Holy Spirit's Interpretation of the New Testament
A Course in Understanding and Acceptance
Regina Dawn Akers
Following on from the strength of *A Course In Miracles*,
NTI teaches us how to experience the love and oneness
of God.
Paperback: 978-1-84694-085-9 ebook: 978-1-78099-083-5

The Message of A Course In Miracles
A translation of the text in plain language
Elizabeth A. Cronkhite
A translation of *A Course in Miracles* into plain, everyday
language for anyone seeking inner peace. The
companion volume, *Practicing A Course In Miracles*,
offers practical lessons and mentoring.
Paperback: 978-1-84694-319-5 ebook: 978-1-84694-642-4

Thinker's Guide to God
Peter Vardy
An introduction to key issues in the philosophy of
religion.
Paperback: 978-1-90381-622-6

Your Simple Path
Find happiness in every step
Ian Tucker
A guide to helping us reconnect with what is really
important in our lives.
Paperback: 978-1-78279-349-6 ebook: 978-1-78279-348-9

365 Days of Wisdom
Daily Messages To Inspire You Through The Year
Dadi Janki
Daily messages which cool the mind, warm the heart
and guide you along your journey.
Paperback: 978-1-84694-863-3 ebook: 978-1-84694-864-0

Body of Wisdom
Women's Spiritual Power and How it Serves
Hilary Hart
Bringing together the dreams and experiences of women
across the world with today's most visionary spiritual
teachers.
Paperback: 978-1-78099-696-7 ebook: 978-1-78099-695-0

Dying to Be Free
From Enforced Secrecy to Near Death to True
Transformation
Hannah Robinson
After an unexpected accident and near-death
experience, Hannah Robinson found herself radically
transforming her life, while a remarkable new insight
altered her relationship with her father a practising
Catholic priest.
Paperback: 978-1-78535-254-6 ebook: 978-1-78535-255-3

The Ecology of the Soul
A Manual of Peace, Power and Personal Growth for Real
People in the Real World
Aidan Walker
Balance your own inner Ecology of the Soul to regain
your natural state of peace, power and wellbeing.
Paperback: 978-1-78279-850-7 ebook: 978-1-78279-849-1

Not I, Not other than I
The Life and Teachings of Russel Williams
Steve Taylor, Russel Williams
The miraculous life and inspiring teachings of one of the
World's greatest living Sages.
Paperback: 978-1-78279-729-6 ebook: 978-1-78279-728-9

On the Other Side of Love
A Woman's Unconventional Journey Towards Wisdom
Muriel Maufroy
When life has lost all meaning, what do you do?
Paperback: 978-1-78535-281-2 ebook: 978-1-78535-282-9

Practicing A Course In Miracles
A Translation of the Workbook in Plain Language and
With Mentoring Notes
Elizabeth A. Cronkhite
The practical second and third volumes of The Plain-
Language *A Course In Miracles*.
Paperback: 978-1-84694-403-1 ebook: 978-1-78099-072-9

Quantum Bliss
The Quantum Mechanics of Happiness, Abundance, and
Health
George S. Mentz
Quantum Bliss is the breakthrough summary of success
and spirituality secrets that customers have been
waiting for.
Paperback: 978-1-78535-203-4 ebook: 978-1-78535-204-1

The Upside Down Mountain
Mags MacKean
A must-read for anyone weary of chasing success and
happiness – one woman's inspirational journey
swapping the uphill slog for the downhill slope.
Paperback: 978-1-78535-171-6 ebook: 978-1-78535-172-3

Your Personal Tuning Fork
The Endocrine System
Deborah Bates
Discover your body's health secret, the endocrine
system, and 'twang' your way to sustainable health!
Paperback: 978-1-84694-503-8 ebook: 978-1-78099-697-4

Readers of ebooks can buy or view any of these bestsellers by clicking on the live link in the title. Most titles are published in paperback and as an ebook. Paperbacks are available in traditional bookshops. Both print and ebook formats are available online.

Find more titles and sign up to our readers' newsletter at
http://www.johnhuntpublishing.com/mind-body-spirit

Follow us on Facebook at
https://www.facebook.com/OBooks/